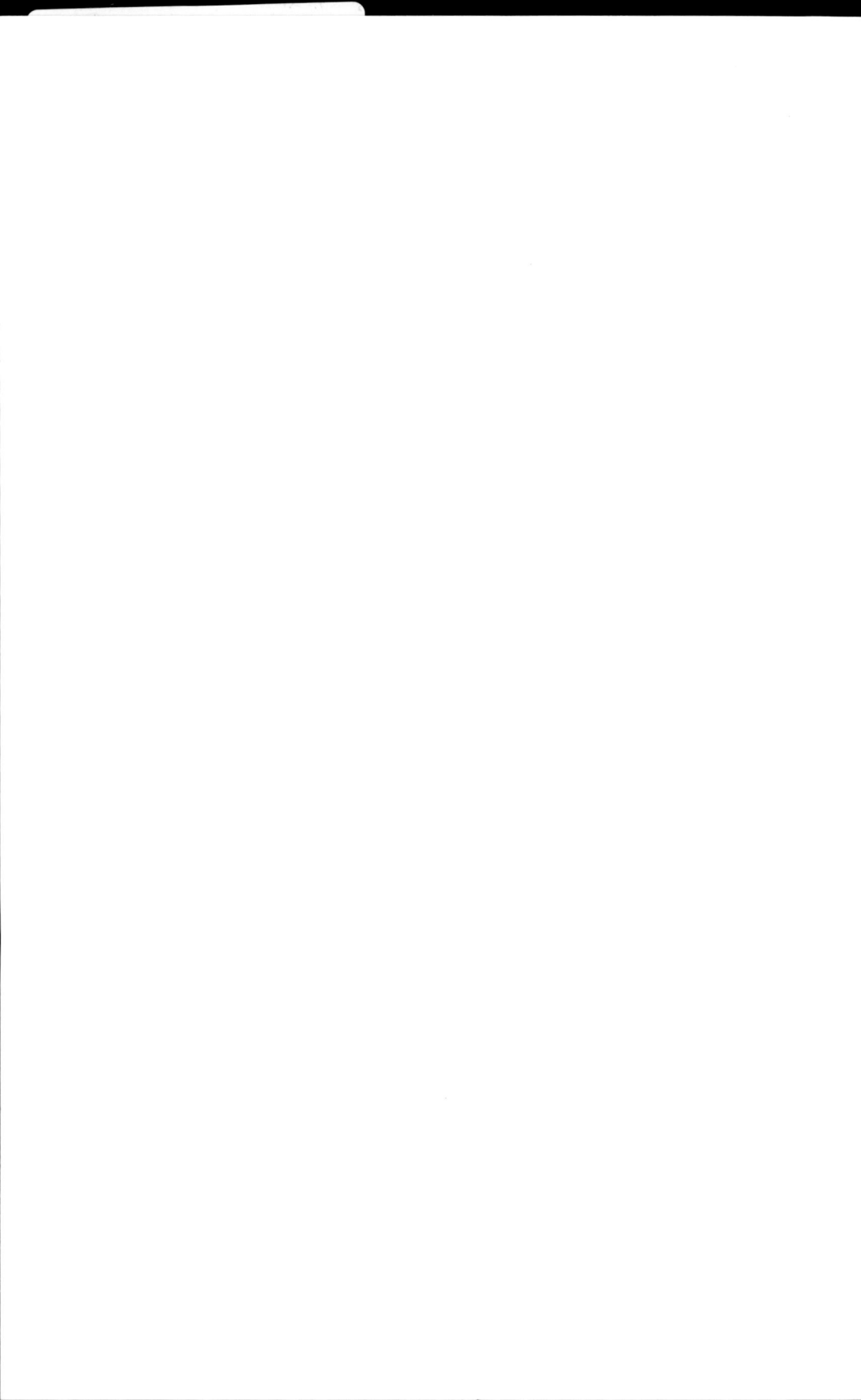

THE
NARROWING

THE
NARROWING

*A Journey Through Anxiety
and the Body*

Dr. Alexandra Shaker

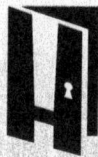

First published in the USA in 2025 by VIKING, an imprint of Penguin Random House LLC

First published in the UK in 2025 by Headline Home An imprint of Headline Publishing Group Limited

1

Cataloguing in Publication Data is available from the British Library

Hardback ISBN 978 1 4722 9561 3
ebook ISBN 978 1 4722 9563 7

Offset in 12.22/18.78pt Granjon LT Std by Jouve (UK), Milton Keynes

Printed and bound in Great Britain by Clays Ltd, Elcograf S.p.A.

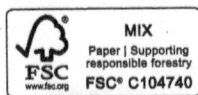

FSC MIX
Paper | Supporting responsible forestry
FSC® C104740

Headline's policy is to use papers that are natural, renewable and recyclable products and made from wood grown in well-managed forests and other controlled sources. The logging and manufacturing processes are expected to conform to the environmental regulations of the country of origin.

Headline Publishing Group Limited
An Hachette UK Company
Carmelite House
50 Victoria Embankment
London EC4Y 0DZ

The authorized representative in the EEA is Hachette Ireland,
8 Castlecourt Centre, Dublin 15, D15 XTP3, Ireland (email: info@hbgi.ie)

www.headline.co.uk
www.hachette.co.uk

All descriptions of my work with former patients are, for the sake of privacy, amalgams of multiple individuals, and all such descriptions have been fully deidentified.

To Houston and Rob

In short, our gentleman became so caught up in reading that he spent his nights reading from dusk till dawn and his days reading from sunrise to sunset, and so with too little sleep and too much reading his brains dried up, causing him to lose his mind.

—Miguel de Cervantes, *Don Quixote*, translated by Edith Grossman

Let me return to the *OED*, where we find that, in sixteenth-century English . . . health is a verb. It might be fun if we could say of our patients, not to mention our loved ones, enemies, even ourselves, that, whatever their sufferings and struggle, "They are now healthing, and carrowsing deepe."

—Muriel Dimen, "Reflections on Cure: or, 'I/Thou/It'"

CONTENTS

AUTHOR'S NOTE

Throughout this book, you'll see that I discuss a good deal of research, and in doing so, I've kept certain criteria in mind. I've addressed long-standing principles of anxiety, and I've sought out recent, high-quality research to reflect the current state of the art—work that is opening up new ways of thinking about, and of treating, anxiety. I've also included some research that is, at the time of this writing, cutting edge—and as such, I've elected to include some findings that have yet to be replicated in the ways that older research has been. In this way, I've tried to situate anxiety in its scientific context while always maintaining an eye toward what is to come. An anxious stance, indeed.

Nonetheless, in thinking through scientific work, we need to keep in mind two fundamental principles: as in all areas of life, (1) correlation does not imply causation, and (2) things change. Research on anxiety is often correlational, meaning that an *association* is found between two things like, say, high levels of anxiety and high levels of impulsivity—so, among people with high levels of anxiety, you tend also to find high levels of impulsivity. Yet these studies cannot demonstrate that one *causes* the other. We should always have the limitations of research in mind in order to put findings in their proper context and, most of all, in order to think about what the research may, functionally, mean in our lives or in the lives of people we care for. And science evolves, as it should, so some of the findings presented here may be read in a different light in the future. Our beliefs about what is true, what is right, what is helpful—they are unstable (again, as they should be). Much as we would like them to be, things often aren't cut and dry. There is, inevitably, tension between what we do know, what we don't know, and what we are just beginning to understand. One could argue that, in fact, anxiety's greatest wisdom and its most devastating consequences both stem from perceiving the infinite depths of our uncertainty.

In the early days of working on this book, I read Maria Popova's *Figuring,* a gorgeous history of art, science, and love. Popova quotes the great environmental activist and prolific writer Rachel Carson, who suggested that writing should contain "the magic combination of factual knowledge and deeply felt emotional response." It is exactly this joining that, in my heart of hearts, I have tried (humbly!) to bring to my work. I find that it is in this very meeting point that we can feel deeply, and in doing so, come to know ourselves anew. Facts, data, information alone—they are essential, yet they aren't enough. They must exist together, with feeling. This book is deeply felt, to my core, and I hope that you feel it too.

ANXIETY AND ME:
ANXIETY AS POTENTIAL

I am afraid to own a Body—
I am afraid to own a Soul—
Profound—precarious Property—
Possession, not optional—

—Emily Dickinson

nxiety gnaws at me more days than not. I'm well acquainted
with the definitions, the symptom checklists, the medication
options, the breathing techniques. I'm a clinical psychologist.
I benefit from this knowledge, I see the visible good it can do, yet I'm
enraged by its limitations. Despite it all, anxiety has a way of creeping in around the edges, and it remains a fixed presence in my life—
lurking, dislocating other experiences, taking up my time.

It is often said that research is me-search. Studying anxiety, treating
it clinically, and writing about it is, for me, both a personal and a
professional endeavor. I've struggled with anxiety for as long as I can
remember, and I suspect that it will remain with me always. Anxiety
is, in every manifestation of it I've ever seen, as much a carnal problem

as it is a cerebral one. I know all too well the sinking, burning feeling that envelops me when anxiety creeps in, and the accompanying self-recrimination for not being able to stave it off from the start. Panic seems to invade every muscle, every vein, every cell. My heart races, my appetite disappears. Then: fear of what could be, probabilities ignored. Worry about making a catastrophic mistake, so devastating that the guilt would consume me and recovery would be impossible. A wish to do away with worry completely, alongside an excruciatingly high bar for certainty—an unreachable bar, really. Certainty, for me, would mean achieving a miraculous state of shatterproof confidence that disaster will not befall me or the people I love.

Anxiety is in our brains, our blood, our hearts, and our guts—it is undeniably corporeal. It makes itself known in our particular worries and fears, but also in our DNA, in our blood pressure, in our heart rates, our digestion. Even the word "anxiety" points toward its bodily manifestations. My favorite definition of anxiety, from the *Dictionary of Untranslatables*, explains, "The term 'anxiety' is etymologically related to that of 'narrowness,' or 'tightening.'" This is among the most experientially accurate descriptions of anxiety that I've encountered. Anxiety is always of the body and of the mind. It brings about a particular narrowness and tightening of thought, yes, but also of the sympathetic nervous system kicking into gear, as the brain takes in extra oxygen, the blood vessels constrict, the heart races, and the guts halt. To feel as though there isn't enough air in the room, to be stuck in a circular, claustrophobic, devastating thought, to have the sense that your veins have been pumped full of terror—it's a certain kind of hell.

Anxiety is among the most human of experiences. It is built into us from the start, and has been, seemingly, forever. For this reason, we find it, over the course of history, explored, taken apart, and revealed, far beyond the bounds of psychology and psychiatry. I suspect that anxiety will always occupy an uneasy position in our minds, being at once a fact of life and a category of diagnoses, as much an existential problem as a behavioral or biological one. Anxiety disorders are defined, yes, and not all of us will experience them as such—but anxiety is also part of being alive. At its core, anxiety shows us that biological and existential questions aren't so far apart, and that they are in constant conversation with each other. Anxiety is medical and it is mental—and it is so much more.

Psychology exists at the crossroads of the arts and the sciences. It stretches between empirical research and human feeling, yet it does so with difficulty. Today, in our attempts to understand the forces that underpin our experiences, we are easily seduced by reductiveness— of seeing the arts and the sciences as opposing forces. Yet psychology refuses to be relegated to the realm of either the biological or discarnate. The body, in all its corporeal ooze and its transcendence, is this way too. Our bodies seem to know things before we are able to put words to them. A headache, a stomachache, a racing heart precede a thought. A gut instinct prevents disaster. Even the most carnal aspects of human experience—that our bodies are imperfect, that pain and illness are inevitable, that our organs eventually cease to function altogether—neither exclude nor fully explain the intangible ones—that we experience connectedness and joy beyond measure, that we have, and sometimes lose, hope, that we love. Rather, they work in tandem. In this way, the body teaches us about ourselves and our place in the world.

This book has been on my mind for many years, and from a range of vantage points. I came to psychology somewhat indirectly. I studied comparative literature first and moved my way into the sciences little by little. I am forever grateful for the way that this path unfolded—it has helped me to think about the sphere of psychology as a broad one, and as one that benefits profoundly from cross-pollination with other disciplines (it turns out that classes on comparative literature tend to take far more interest in Freud than the average course in psychology does).

My graduate training in psychology took place in New York City, beginning in 2009. I see in retrospect how fortunate I am for both of these elements—the place and the time. I was taught to look at human experience and psychotherapy from (at least) two perspectives, a circumstance that is increasingly hard to come by in higher education, which is becoming more and more ideologically divided. There is a tendency within psychology to adhere strictly, to cling, really, to one school of thought or another when it comes to mental illness and its treatment—for instance, working within a cognitive approach, or a psychoanalytic one. Is anxiety, say, the fault of a lack of reasonable thinking? Or does it reflect internal conflict? Is it treated by identifying and correcting irrational thought patterns or by understanding long-standing family dynamics? I find that this closes doors, and it narrows the mind.

I was most influenced by my teachers and supervisors who worked from a psychodynamic perspective (typically associated with Sigmund Freud)—that is, to consider both conscious and unconscious forces in our lives, and to pay close attention to how early development influences us. But also, I was taught to think from a cognitive behavioral point of view, which focuses on the relationship between feelings, thoughts, and behaviors, and on practical techniques for symptom management. My teachers traversed these theoretical perspectives and they traversed generations, and I am deeply indebted to them for their sensitivity and depth, and for their wisdom—they taught me the power in both of these perspectives. Over time, I came to see psychology as a field that moves forward when we look not only inward but outward—when we are curious.

Psychology is, then, a field that defies strict delineation—and psychological questions offer us an opportunity to think through our most essential human struggles through the wisdom of multiple traditions. In understanding anxiety as biological and social, historical and intergenerational, we can draw from a newly wide world of experience, one that more fully reflects our reality. We can learn about anxiety, and then about resilience, from current research in biology, just as we can from our family trees or from literature of past centuries. It is at these crossroads that some of the most exciting work happens. Science, at its heart and at its best, is meant to illuminate the world, and the world is anything but tidy. We look to science, rightly, for invaluable, indeed life-changing information—and we look elsewhere for communion and wisdom. I've found more solace in my favorite works of literature than from any peer-reviewed paper. This isn't the fault of science—it's that I am human. If a person considering a career in psychology were to ask me what to major in, or how best to prepare for their studies, I would tell them to read, and widely.

It is in this spirit that I reach beyond the usual confines of discussions about anxiety—that is, beyond the symptom checklists, or going to sleep with your phone in the other room, and beyond Western culture's current fixation on positivity, in order to offer the sort of expansiveness of thought that I've found most helpful for myself and that I hope to impart upon others. I find that in this way, anxiety can be rooted in a sense of history and human connection that helps us to see its meaning, its many dimensions, rather than being exclusively a thorn in our side, or even a source of suffering. There are no easy answers, but there is awesome potential. The language of anxiety is neurology and psychology and biology and physiology and philosophy and sociology and anthropology and literature and poetry.

Carl Jung wrote: "To the psychotherapist, whose special field lies just in this crucial sphere of the interaction of mind and body, it seems highly probable that the psychic and the physical are not two independent parallel processes, but are essentially connected through reciprocal action, although the exact nature of this relationship is still completely outside our experience." In this book, we will trace anxiety's path through the body. We will look at the interplay between our physiology and our minds—and we will look further. Our bodies are a constant reminder of our humanity. Within their confines, we are faced with our potential, and, too, with our mortality. You notice an oncoming headache, or feel the blood rush out of your face or your heart begin to race—and there it is: proof of life and its limits, the seeds of anxiety.

Rather than being prescriptive, my hope is that in seeing anxiety through a multidimensional lens, in seeing anxiety with depth, we can, together, find what anxiety has to teach us about being alive—without losing sight of certain truths. Most of all, that life includes pain. That there are no hacks that will truly rid you of anxiety—and that ultimately, this is OK. We can be strong and fragile at the same time, always mortal, but still probably OK, and in the end, we don't get to know most things for sure. As with much of life, the things that most trouble us, our own stumbling blocks, are also the things that tend to be most valuable to work through. It is resilience, not cure, that we should be striving for.

I try throughout to show you my own uncertainties and ambivalences, and the uncertainties that remain even when we are surrounded by data. I don't try to fit a square peg into a round hole. Though it is often uncomfortable, we can feel and even believe more than one thing at a time—and to acknowledge these ambivalences and uncertainties are their own kind of resistance against anxiety.

At every turn, I've tried to bring together layers of meaning—from research on the ways that anxiety manifests in our bodies, to the ways that the symbolism of our bodies can shed light on our inner lives and can help us to cultivate strength and steadiness. I've interviewed a range of experts in fields including psychology, psychiatry, neuroscience, neurobiology, and economics—because I believe that understanding anxiety requires a wide lens. Here, form follows function—and from chapter to chapter, I integrate fields of study while moving through the body, from the brain to the blood to the heart to the gut. I look at the ways that each of these areas in the body gives anxiety its shape and texture—from the thoughts and fears that play out in our brains to the sensations that pop up in our guts. I believe that it is in understanding our histories (personal and shared) and our bodies in tandem that we find a way through anxiety. After all, anxiety exists most potently in our daily lives, in the world as it is, not in a textbook or a laboratory.

ↂ

When I began graduate school, I bought my first copy of the *Diagnostic and Statistical Manual of Mental Disorders* (DSM) for a course on adult psychopathology. The chapter titles include things like "Mood Disorders" and "Anxiety Disorders," and at the time, I felt like I was holding a powerful book, one that might contain the secrets to questions I was struggling to articulate. Looking back, these might have been questions like: Is this worry too much? Why do I feel stuck in these ways?

It works like this: according to the DSM, to be given a particular diagnosis—say, generalized anxiety disorder (GAD) or obsessive-compulsive disorder (OCD), you need to meet a particular set of criteria. Some criteria are essential to the diagnosis, whereas others are optional. So, for instance, OCD can be diagnosed with either obsessions or compulsions—both aren't required. And some criteria have time requirements too—for instance, in the case of GAD, some symptoms must have been occurring for at least six months. In this way, the DSM draws lines around collections of symptoms to arrive at discrete diagnoses (and most of all, it is used to bill insurance companies for services).

As I worked my way through this book (studying obsessively, which, despite reading about obsessionality, did not occur to me at the time) and soon after was in the position of evaluating new patients to determine a diagnosis and develop a treatment plan, I saw firsthand how flawed this system is, how profoundly limited in its capacity to describe human experience, and how it is entirely devoid of the curative magic that I was wishing for. Rather, my anxiety was unchanged from reading the DSM, despite having done so with the utmost care and in its entirety. I saw in the DSM bits of myself scattered across sections—a bit of panic, a bit of obsessionality, a lot of worrying. In retrospect, I think this is true for most people. Rather than fitting cleanly into categories, with reflection we can observe in ourselves varying degrees of experiences that shift throughout our days, our weeks, and the stages we move through in our lives.

Although our current diagnostic system suggests that mental illnesses can be cleanly divided and labeled, there is a great deal of overlap among diagnoses, and people often don't fit conveniently within existing categories. This plagues scientific research, which holds clarity in the highest esteem, yet it is difficult to study discrete entities when they aren't, in fact, discrete.

When it comes to the diagnosis of anxiety disorders, it is crucial to remember that anxiety is an experience that exists on a continuum—one that includes the anxieties of everyday life, those that are inevitably part of being human. It is, for instance, entirely healthy to experience worry and sadness; you would be hard-pressed to find anyone who hasn't (and if you did, I suspect that you would find other sorts of problems instead). The continuum shifts into the realm of mental illness when it interferes with one's life and becomes a source of suffering. There is a big difference between, say, sometimes worrying about a family conflict and worrying so often and so deeply that you sleep poorly, feel irritable and restless, and struggle to perform at work. And although diagnostic tools are useful in establishing a common language for the purposes of treatment and research, they are a kind of shorthand. Because anxiety fits squarely within the spheres of both health and illness, it can be slippery—it has a remarkable way of escaping the confines of traditional diagnoses and classifications.

The history of our current diagnostic system, and really, of nosology itself (that is, the ways in which diseases of all kinds are classified), dates back to ancient times. Somewhat more recently, in the seventeenth century, Robert Burton composed his wild, meandering *The Anatomy of Melancholy*. Burton was interested in the particulars of people's pain. He collected their anecdotal experiences alongside the works of medical scholars. Together, they form one of the most remarkable descriptions of the sorts of troubles that emerge in our internal lives that exists today, no matter that this text is some four hundred years old. In his catalogue of symptoms of melancholy, Burton includes "palpitation of the heart, short breath, plenty of humidity in the stomach, heaviness of heart & heartache." Although our diagnostic systems have evolved considerably since the seventeenth century, Burton reminds us: for as much as we wish to cleanly divide our experiences, different kinds of pain bleed together.

There is now a great deal of scholarship and clinical research devoted to nosology in the context of mental illness. Central to this work is the question of whether a dimensional or a categorical model is best suited to mental illness. Our current diagnostic system is categorical, meaning that illnesses are divided into discrete, seemingly neat categories like generalized anxiety disorder or panic disorder. On the other hand, in a dimensional model, the idea is to work instead with symptom dimensions—for instance, restlessness or trouble sleeping. In this way, symptoms are looked at on a continuum, and the inconsistencies in the ways in which mental illness presents itself in different individuals are more clearly identified. So, in the most

basic form, instead of two people who are having qualitatively different experiences both receiving a broad-strokes diagnosis of generalized anxiety disorder, each would instead have a profile of sorts,
reflecting the particulars of their individual experiences. One might,
for instance, be high in worry and irritability but low in restlessness
and in difficulty sleeping, whereas another person could be high in
irritability, worry, restlessness, and difficulty sleeping. These sorts of
differences could have meaningful implications for treatment.

The Hierarchical Taxonomy of Psychopathology system (known
as HiTOP) is an effort to create a system of diagnosis for mental illness within a dimensional framework. Researchers at a range of insti-
tutions are in an ongoing process of honing this model for use in
clinical and research settings. Essentially, the lowest level of the
model is made up of symptoms and signs (whereas symptoms are
reported, for instance, "I feel tense all the time," signs are observed,
for instance, "patient tapped their foot and fidgeted throughout the
session"); the highest level of the model is an overall psychopathology
score that shows the severity of the individual's illness. Research suggests that in addition to being useful in clinical practice, the HiTOP
model is also more reflective of the genetic underpinnings of mental
illness than is our current diagnostic system. For me, and I think for
many people, there is an intuitive appeal to the concept of a dimensional diagnostic system. It *feels* truer that my experience or yours, all
of ours, would be better captured, better described, in this way. A
dimensional diagnostic system, one in which there is room for a
greater deal of individual difference, of human specificity, strikes me
as more sensitive, more human. It is only natural to try to force our
struggles into clear categories, to lay them out just so, with the hopes

of comprehending and resolving them. But again, most often, things aren't so clear.

 formats≈

We tend to view anxiety as a problem of the individual, a matter of, briefly put, worrying too much, and a problem whose causes and cures should be discussed and delivered privately. And the work of treating individuals' anxiety is important, vital, even. It is work that I've done as a therapist and as a patient, work that I believe in deeply. But anxiety stretches far beyond our private experiences. It is a vast force, with entrenched social and biological roots. Today, we are living amid undeniable precarity—in precarious bodies, on a precarious planet, at the mercy of precarious health systems and economies and international relations, and under the pressures of a seemingly infinite flow of information. Disaster seems not only possible but close at hand, and our collective anxiety has become uncontainable. Studies from 2020 and 2021 show a striking upsurge in mortality salience—which is to say, collectively we have death on our minds. As recently as 2020, researchers identified sobering increases in anxiety, depression, and thoughts of suicide (in the United States, reports of anxiety or depression have just about quadrupled over the past two years, and similar studies from the UK show anxiety and depression nearly doubling). We are raw with the knowledge that, for better or for worse, the future is unknowable. We are being reminded every day, abruptly and painfully, that anxiety can find its way to us all, and that it casts a long shadow.

We are talking about anxiety in public. There is a palpable shift in the air toward normalizing discussion of our vulnerabilities, and toward finding meaningful connections in the midst of our pain. It's not only that we are in urgent need of looking at anxiety with depth and nuance (though that is certainly true)—it's also that, now, we want to. And on some level, we've been talking about this for centuries, albeit in other words. Anxiety has been at the heart of our creative and intellectual lives throughout history—with scores of our most significant thinkers wrestling with the complex connections between mind and body—from the works of Stoic philosophers to Robert Burton's *The Anatomy of Melancholy* to Freud's writing on the relationship between trauma and anxiety.

The history of anxiety's place in psychology and psychiatry is long and winding. Anxiety has, at different points in history, been conceptualized as bodily, mental, or both, and even as a moral problem. Looking back to the fifth century BCE, when Hippocratic medicine was taking shape, anxiety was often seen as a lack of internal strength. In *Anxiety: A Short History*, sociologist Allan V. Horwitz writes: "Anxiety in the ancient world was more likely to be seen as a sign of moral failure than as a medical dysfunction."

A few centuries later, humoral theory began to drive much of Western medicine. Humoral theory was centered around the principle that imbalances in the body lead to problems of health of all kinds, and in turn, that bodily balance is the way to address illness. Treatment for anxiety was in the vein of what we might now call changes in lifestyle—for instance, as Horwitz explains, "changes in diet, exercise, sexual activity, and sleep." Herbal remedies were at times prescribed, as described in *The Anatomy of Melancholy*: "Marigold is much approved against Melancholy, and often used therefore in our ordinary broth, as good against this and many other diseases. . . . And because the spleen and blood are often misaffected in melancholy, I may not omit Endive, Succory, Dandelion . . . which cleanse the blood." In the context of modern science and today's constantly shifting treatment options, it can be difficult to appreciate how long-lasting principles of humoral theory were in the history of medicine; but in fact, they remained at the center of Western medicine for centuries.

Beliefs about the nature of mental illness—both its causes and how to treat it—changed in the seventeenth century, at which point physicians began to attribute anxiety (among other conditions) to the body in a new way, looking to problems with the nervous system and the brain in particular. In this period, the broad term "nervous disorders" came into use and included what we now call anxiety disorders. Treatment for anxiety continued to emphasize lifestyle factors but also included substances like opium.

At the end of the nineteenth century, Sigmund Freud, who was trained as a neurologist, began to take interest in the unconscious factors that contribute to mental distress. He was fascinated by anxiety and its causes, and he is known most of all for the development of psychoanalysis, a form of psychotherapy that emphasizes the value of developing insight into one's experiences, often through free association. Over the course of the twentieth century, parallel to the development of psychoanalysis, another kind of treatment for anxiety emerged: behavior therapy. Early on, behavior therapy was applied to forms of anxiety, like phobias. According to the principles of behavior therapy, as renowned expert on anxiety and obsessive compulsive disorder Stanley Rachman explains, "Treatment should promote the extinction of the unadaptive behavior and enhance adaptive behavior." Behavior therapy and psychoanalysis were (and remain) markedly distinct approaches to anxiety, with behavioral approaches focusing on measurable behaviors, and psychoanalysis emphasizing internal, subjective experiences.

In the mid-twentieth century, alongside the development of psychoanalysis and behavior therapy, new psychiatric medications for anxiety were introduced. In the 1950s and '60s, physicians prescribed tranquilizers for anxiety, and they were soon followed by benzodiazepines (a type of medication that is still in use today, like Xanax, and is often prescribed for panic attacks). In the 1980s, selective serotonin reuptake inhibitors (SSRIs; like Prozac, Zoloft, and Lexapro), which were initially aimed at treating depression, also came to be used to treat anxiety disorders, and they remain one of the most commonly used treatments for anxiety disorders today.

Looking back, despite so many advancements in modern science, some things haven't changed. Modern society has yet to outgrow the misconception that anxiety is a moral problem. Most of us have encountered the notion, put upon us by other people (or even as a nagging voice in one's own mind), that anxiety indicates a lack of toughness. And when it comes to humoral theory, although much of it sounds absurd to the modern ear (we no longer think of health in terms of blood and phlegm, black and yellow bile), the principle of balance in day-to-day life remains at the forefront of contemporary conceptions of well-being. In historical efforts to identify causes of anxiety in the nervous system, we see the roots of modern clinical research on anxiety's biological and genetic underpinnings. And both psychodynamic and behavioral therapies, in new iterations, are found around the world in clinical and research settings. We see, then, that anxiety and its treatment are very old problems. It comes as no surprise that despite so many efforts to understand and tame it, anxiety is still in the ascendancy. Estimates from the World Health Organization suggest that in 2019, some 301 million people globally were living with anxiety that reached diagnostic thresholds for an anxiety disorder. Across time and terms, anxiety is a part of us, hardy, and, it seems, unexorcisable.

ᥣᴓ

When we were little, my younger sister, who was around four years old at the time, told our mother that when I learned to read, it "ruined our relationship." Reading felt to me like a way to expand the world. I most loved books like *Harriet the Spy* and *The Baby-Sitters Club* series, which made me feel like children could do big things. But when I was about ten, my interests shifted from stories of children making things happen to stories of children dying tragically, mostly from cancer. I became obsessed with books by Lurlene McDaniel, who had a corner on young adult novels about children and teenagers facing death, usually from terminal illness. I wonder now what my parents made of me reading books with titles like *Six Months to Live, No Time to Cry, Sixteen and Dying*, and *If I Should Die Before I Wake*. I learned the telltale signs of leukemia (unexplained bruises, frequent bloody noses), and, for a time, these stories consumed me. In retrospect, I think perhaps this was my first attempt at understanding my own burgeoning anxiety, and really, my existential terror—most of all, my fears of catastrophe and loss. I was afraid of my parents dying, afraid of going to the dentist, afraid of developing a fatal illness. I was terrified by the inescapable fragility of my body, and of all the ways that the body is never fully knowable. As a teenager, my anxiety, which was often tied up in an overwhelming, unrealistic sense of responsibility for the people in my life, grew. When I was seventeen, I had my first (of many) panic attacks—and, not unusually, as I began to feel my anxiety closing in on me, I became terrified that I was having a heart attack. But even after extensive medical exams confirmed the health of my heart, my anxiety persisted.

The following year, within months of beginning university in New York City, I developed what I (being from a rural area) believed to be spider bites on my torso. A few days later, student health services informed me that I had shingles, likely caused by stress. I began therapy, and at my first appointment, my psychologist recommended that I take yoga classes. She pointed me toward research showing the benefits of yoga and controlled breathing for anxiety management. At that point, I would have done anything she suggested to quell my frequent panic attacks, which left me feeling like my body was utterly vulnerable and entirely out of my control. For a time, I went to classes religiously, at a studio near my dormitory. Each hour began with chanting in Sanskrit as the teacher played the harmonium. Initially, I found this awkward and, frankly, embarrassing; I struggled to keep my eyes closed and to stop myself from fidgeting. But as I learned to put my discomfort aside, I gradually came to find it soothing, and those early minutes of each class became a reliable source of calm. As it turns out, neuroscience explains this—chanting, singing, and other forms of music are known to reduce anxiety as we experience it in our minds and our bodies.

17

Though my understanding of the complex relationship between my anxiety and my body was just beginning to unfold, this felt like the first successful step I'd taken to temper and transform the power my anxiety had over me. I wasn't cured, not by a long shot, but little by little, my body began to feel more like an ally and less like a source of potential disaster. The beating of my heart could, in the right light, be a sign of my vitality instead of my fear.

By the time I reached my early twenties, I was keenly aware that, even with psychotherapy and medication, even with yoga and the full gamut of practical techniques, anxiety would be a part of my life, always within me, and, for better and for worse, it has shaped me. As I began my clinical training, I was quickly immersed in the many ways in which our bodies can be the sites and expressions of our pain—from panic to health anxiety to substance misuse to self-injury to binging and purging—and living within them can feel unbearable. I see the threads of anxiety deeply embedded in my life, stitched into my body, sometimes taking up a great deal of space, and sometimes receding into the background. And though my fears of loss and uncertainty have shape-shifted over the years, in many ways, at their core, they remain the same.

Everyone has their pain, whether you know about it or not. As a therapist, this becomes both essential to keep in mind and impossible to forget—you are reminded every day that the surface conceals histories and wounds beyond your imagination. But in a strange twist of logic, as soon as I began graduate school to study clinical psychology, I got the sense that it would be an embarrassment, a source of shame even, to have any personal skin in the game of psychology, as though there could be some "pure" entry into the field, having nothing to do with my own struggles. In spite of this, little by little, it became clear that we all had our reasons. There were students who had suffered terrible losses, and others who knew depression intimately or who had painful family histories. Nobody becomes a clinical psychologist out of academic interest or altruism alone. As a particularly insightful professor would often remind us: "The bigger the front, the bigger the back"—which is to say: when we make massive efforts, whether they be working toward a degree or conveying a tough-as-nails exterior, you can be sure that there is another story beneath the surface. And in the end, those reasons expose themselves, whether you mean for them to or not. My interest in studying psychology—and I suspect this was true for many of my fellow students—was complicated. It was a decision that grew out of genuine academic curiosity and aspiration, out of a sincere hope to be of use to other people, and, too, out of the things that plagued me in my own life. There my anxiety was, fixed firmly within my body and my mind. And now, with the wisdom of some degree of hindsight, my decision to share aspects of my own experiences is one that I've made with great care. Traditionally, psychologists are trained to share very little information about themselves—to do so only minimally, and only if necessary. This is based on the premise that we can, in this way, become a blank slate for our patients. With much consideration, I've come to feel that to write deeply about anxiety without speaking to my own experiences would be inauthentic, dishonest—indeed, I think that readers would feel it. I've come to see my personal and professional perspectives on anxiety as working hand in hand, and I believe that I can offer something more useful, and, I hope, more profound, from this place—as a psychologist, yes, but also as a mother, a partner, a friend. We are all human—nobody is exempt. And I find that one of our most vital instincts, one that we can see all around us, is to make our struggles into something useful.

As I approached the completion of my seemingly endless graduate studies, I went on a weeklong, much awaited vacation to Iceland (as was the fashion at the time). It was a joyful, exhilarating holiday, but it also presaged a period of the most crushing anxiety I had experienced in my life, followed by depression. Upon returning home to my usual routines, rumination (those miserable, repetitive, circular worries that are often a desperate attempt at problem-solving) took hold. Anxiety is insidious—it expands into spaces you didn't notice before. What had previously been a subtle, easily disregarded instinct became a gut feeling writ large: something is not right.

Now I see it clearly. Away from home, with the time and space to think outside of my day-to-day, I felt like I could breathe. With a renewed sense of motion and expansiveness, I allowed myself to imagine new possibilities that reached beyond the confines of what I had thought my professional life would consist of. As my years of training in psychology were coming to a close, I began to feel suffocated by the decades looming ahead of me. I had pushed forward along a clear-cut career path, one whose predictability and structure had initially been a comfort to me, but I had left parts of myself behind. I was horrified that I had embarked on a plan for my life before fully understanding what it would mean—and feared that I had made an awful, irreparable mistake. And though I knew then as I know now that my work in psychology could take many forms, this freedom felt entirely abstract to me. The kind of conflict I'm describing isn't particularly unusual—we've all heard stories of these sorts of misgivings, or navigated them ourselves—but to me, it felt like a shameful secret. When I heard friends talking about their career "pivots," it sounded like a point of pride, an indication of open-mindedness and even entrepreneurialism—so millennial and light. I envied the empathy that they had for themselves. I know myself to be a solid person—I do what I say I'll do. I finish what I start. I'm trustworthy, responsible. My uncertainties felt like a negation of all that. What ate away at me most of all was that for years there had been whispers of doubt in my mind that I had pushed past. I had put one foot in front of the other and worked like a demon to get where I was. In so many ways, it would have been easier to continue along the same path regardless, to hope that things would shift on their own, that my doubts would fade into the background. But I knew that this would be a betrayal, and that I would need to find a way to reincorporate the parts of myself that I had unwittingly abandoned. It was thrilling, and, as is often the case, terrifying too. It was the first time in years that I had allowed myself to entertain a change in my plans or my desires, and it felt like an emergency.

Over the course of a few weeks, I became consumed with worry and doubt about all the ways that I might make any number of highly improbable catastrophic mistakes. I double-, triple-checked my work. Fear of a hair straightener left plugged in during a weekend at my grandmother's led to an extra four hours in heavy traffic when I insisted that we double back. Any bit of free time was consumed with a replaying of the past week's events, most of all the moments in which I wished I had done things differently. I felt like I was suffocating. I would try to envisage all possible outcomes and identify strategies to prevent these unlikely disasters. Against my better judgment, I fell into seeing the depth and extent of this worrying as protective, preventative, and preparative, as though bypassing this step would be a devil-may-care invitation to calamity. My heart raced. I struggled to sleep and lost my appetite. My muscles felt tense and my hands were shaky. My uncertainties felt heavy and awful. I could barely put words to them within my own mind, much less speak them aloud. I berated myself, questioning decisions I had made, and I felt ashamed of my uncertainty as I struggled to see that changing one's mind is not a crime. That awful narrowness took hold.

It wasn't long before depression set in. This is not uncommon—anxiety and depression often coexist. And while there is anxiety that ignites you and keeps you on your toes, moving toward a goal, anxiety that dips into depression is another thing altogether. Research suggests that nearly half the people who meet criteria for generalized anxiety disorder will also meet criteria for major depressive disorder, and some studies show an even higher rate of overlap. This is not to say that anxiety necessarily causes depression, but that the two hang together. It *feels* causal, as though little by little, constant anxiety wears you down, and eventually depression takes hold. The brain can only sustain high levels of anxiety for so long.

That year, I felt most useful, most alive, during the hours I spent working on an inpatient unit for people with severe eating disorders. There, amid so much loss and anger and fear, was the agony of the body and all that it contains. The anxiety was palpable and entirely unavoidable—and so, too, were questions of the brain, the blood, the heart, and the guts, as they exist in our bodies and in all that they stand for. There were physiological crises of, among other things, cardiac status and nutrition—and there were existential questions too. What does it mean to think reasonably? What do we pass on to our children, be it through our blood lines or our environments? How can we find space for connection and even love in the midst of chaos? And what happens when we relinquish control?

Today, I see that that period was an inevitable, necessary impasse. I felt caught between seemingly opposing states—anxious yet bold, at a loss yet determined, and unable to see how to embody these states simultaneously. But fundamentally, I knew that I was not actually trapped. I knew that my anxiety and depression were temporary states with imperfect but good-enough remedies, and that the world is large and exists outside the confines of my brain, my body. That if I looked for the thread, I would find it. It was a reckoning. I smelled possibility.

಄

Between hope and dread, there is friction. On one hand, there is so much promise, so much solace to be found in all that science is teaching us, in all that we are learning about the workings of our bodies. But despite our best efforts, dread is there too, lurking, often within arm's reach, and the proximity of the two can be disorienting. Most of us tend to push aside feelings that we fear we will not be able to cope with. We avoid them, sometimes for years on end, without knowing we are doing so. But nothing just disappears (Freud famously wrote about "the return of the repressed"). When it comes to anxiety, it is in facing the dread head-on that the hope begins to feel stronger.

I want to understand how our anxieties can control our bodies, how our bodies can contain or rebel against the output of our minds, and ultimately, how we can learn to transform this fundamental tenet of living into something that won't hold us back. When anxiety takes my breath away, I want to turn it on its head and draw upon the energy buried beneath it. Rather than falling into distraction and emotional paralysis, I will be nimble and capacious.

Which brings me to the perennial question: How do you get out of your own way?

Without clear, effective, and practical methods to reduce anxiety, we get nowhere. I humbly bow down to the many treatment options that exist, behavioral and medicinal. And I partake in them. We've grown accustomed to pragmatic approaches to treating anxiety, like workbooks, list making, habit tracking, and so on. The promise of practical tactics is seductive, because when we are in pain, we seek relief. Let me be absolutely clear: to treat symptoms first is important, even lifesaving. Research consistently supports a range of methods to reduce symptoms of anxiety—from exercise to breathing techniques. These strategies are vital—because when you are suffering, symptom relief needs to come first. Without it, there is no room to think. With the return of some semblance of calm, a calm as much of body as of mind, it becomes possible to move forward. But short-term symptom relief alone provides only transient improvement, and to allow the conversation about anxiety to end with practical strategies leaves a great deal unspoken. They are useful, yet they are not, in the end, enough. Despite so many scientific advances, and despite more and more access to information, we have not outrun our oldest terrors. All the evidence points the same way: we are more afraid, more alone, and more lost.

Anxiety is a felt state of emergency in the absence of an actual emergency. It leads to something I've come to think of as chronic emergency confusion. This plays out quite literally at times—a recent study found that in the United States alone, over the course of one year there were 1.2 million emergency room visits and $42.3 billion spent on health care due to anxiety. And these numbers precede 2020. In my case, this might take the shape of becoming consumed with whether a question that I just remembered I forgot to ask my doctor three years ago could lead to my untimely death, rather than truly disastrous problems like, for example, climate change. In this way, anxiety reorders the importance of things. It distorts likelihoods and feeds preoccupation about hypotheticals (like, say, whether the fact that my friend hasn't responded to my text message could mean that they have suffered a medical emergency alone in their home and can't get to the phone) or things well beyond the bounds of human control, and it detracts from the mental space we need to engage in meaningful actions in the present. Whether you face a real or perceived threat, and even when we know better, bodily systems engage to handle an emergency.

So, I ask myself—will I be undone by uncertainty, or will I accept that there is no choice but to live within its dominion? To what degree will I fight for the illusion of control? Or can I come to terms with the chaos and unknowability that defines the human condition? Anxiety operates at a different volume for each of us, depending on brain chemistry, context, and life experience. To eliminate it entirely would threaten survival: it alerts us to mortal danger. And even in the absence of life-threatening situations, a degree of anxiety can be a strength, insofar as it can contribute to productive thought and action. I've benefited many times from attempting to evade uncertainty—by not letting things go unnoticed and by checking things twice. I was the student who proofread every assignment carefully, the employee who stayed late to make sure that *i*'s were dotted and *t*'s were crossed. Because we live in a world that tends to reward precisely this sort of anxiety with good grades and professional accolades and promotions, the line between healthy, useful anxiety and pathological anxiety can blur. Everyone worries sometimes, but not everyone is tortured by their thoughts; most of us are, on some level, afraid of loss and human fallibility, but most people don't think about it all day. To feel as though you are constantly, uncontrollably spinning among your fears is a problem. Is this sweating the beginning of a heart attack? Is this headache indicative of stress, or a brain tumor? To put a finer point on it, why is it so difficult for some to tolerate the relative mystery of the inside of our own organs, of whatever may be lurking in our veins? Anxiety is often characterized by anticipation of future distress or despair. But as I was once wisely reminded, "suffering does not require rehearsal." For those of us who are, for genetic, environmental, and at times unknowable reasons, susceptible, anxiety becomes a persistent intruder, logic be damned.

Over the years, I have become personally and professionally transfixed by the particular interruptions that anxiety brings about. I have seen lives defined by them and experienced them acutely myself.

Now, whole cultures and communities seem to thrum with anxiety. What would it be like if our thoughts didn't sometimes feel so toxic? How might we live our lives if our minds could wander about, even when things are hard, rather than catching so often on worry and doubt? If we could pump our veins full of vigor instead of dread? If our interests (which are really desires) could remain in place even when we are afraid, instead of being shut out by thoughts of catastrophe or by our ultimate vulnerability? If we could trust our guts, relinquish control, allow ourselves to be defiant? If we could create a boundary, a gate, between ourselves and our thoughts? And I see that it is exactly that which feels lost in the throes of anxiety—vitality, curiosity, nerve, a freedom of mind and of body—that will be the bridge out. Brain, blood, heart, guts—they are what resilience is made of.

When I began to resurface from the depths of my anxiety and depression in the closing stretch of my twenties, there was something new in my relationship with my own body. Its fragility had always terrified me, but there was a new awareness of its robustness, its strength, the things it could confront and overcome. The anxiety that felt like a fire burning within myself, a perpetual emergency—I came to it as a newly plastic force, one that I might learn to shape. I was scared, yes, but I felt the warmth of rebellion too.

ᘖ

I used to believe that although there were and are an infinite number of things I don't understand or know how to remedy, there must be someone, somewhere, who does. I don't believe this anymore. There is no perfect antidote—all we have is trying, and each other. You get up and try again. Resilience frames our view of the past and the future, and resilience can be found in surprising places.

There is a growing body of evidence that it is possible to change the brain and the ways it functions through practices like psychotherapy and meditation. And research is unpacking the impact of everything from social support to spirituality on the development of emotional resilience. These findings are deeply encouraging because they are a reminder that despite anxiety's physiological components, we have an enormous capacity to dust ourselves off and start again. You can literally change your mind. We depend on our resilience more in difficult times, and it's a cornerstone of our psychological health that has been tested in recent years. For most of us, it's an iterative process of looking honestly at our vulnerabilities and responding to them with persistence and with an appreciation for the complexities of living. To cultivate resilience is to explore the edges of yourself—the things you can tolerate comfortably and the things you can just barely stand. Even in the best of times, life is hard. In the words of the renowned Buddhist teacher Sharon Salzberg, "Some things just hurt."

In the brain, between neurons, there is a microscopic space called the synaptic cleft. Here, messages are transmitted from one neuron to another, as neurotransmitters like serotonin and dopamine move from one place to the next. I like to picture the synaptic cleft when I think about cultivating space between myself and my anxiety. I imagine sitting there, tucked into my own brain, as though I were between thoughts, allowing space to increase and time to pass, instead of succumbing to a deluge of worry and doubt. Instead of pushing back, you settle in and let go. Ultimately, to be resilient is to be at home with yourself.

I know now that anxiety is a matter of boundaries, thresholds, and limits. How do you establish boundaries between yourself and others, and between yourself and your thoughts? How do you control what you let in and what you keep out? What are the limits of this control, of power, and of responsibility? What is your threshold for risk, for distress, for uncertainty? How do you approach the past, and its legacy in your body and your mind, and how do you think about the future? These are questions at the heart of our existence, and what I have seen clinically and in my own life is that our answers to them can define us. Anxiety asks, every step of the way: Where is the line?

In Roman mythology, Janus, who is depicted with one face looking toward the future and another toward the past, is the god of doorways and passages. He is also the god of dualities and new beginnings. In Roman cities, Janus gates were said to be open during periods of war and closed during periods of peace. In Janus himself, and in the mythology of the origins of the world, we see embodied the dualities, the painful paradoxes, that shape our lives:

> Some say that Darkness was first, and from Darkness sprang Chaos. From a union between Darkness and Chaos sprang Night, Day, Erebus, and the Air.
>
> From a union between Night and Erebus sprang Doom, Old Age, Death, Murder, Continence, Sleep, Dreams, Discord, Misery, Vexation, Nemesis, Joy, Friendship, Pity, the Three Fates, and the Three Hesperides.

Life is made of beginnings and endings, of limits, of pain and joy, beauty and ugliness—there is no other way.

Now, I see Janus as my god of anxiety too. I imagine my synaptic clefts as Janus gates—as transformational spaces between one thing and the next, where anxiety can become potential and where resilience is born in those expandable spaces in my own mind. I like to imagine that with practice, I will remember, more often and with greater ease, that in spite of any efforts of mine, chaos is all around.

I look forward, I look back. The gates are open, the gates are closed. I am at war, I am at peace. I try, I try again. I lose the thread, I find it. Stubborn and serpentine, anxiety weaves itself into the most elemental ways that we relate to ourselves and to others. A perceived state of emergency. A problem of emphasis and extent. A matter of trust. A question of reason. A wish for control. It is there in our bodies, in the brain, the blood, the heart, and the guts. It is mine and yours, whether we like it or not. There is no cure nor any complete recovery. I'm standing at the gate, always looking backward and always looking forward. But I'm still here, and I'm home.

Part I

BRAIN

1.

ATTENTION

And what was the hope? That all
shadows of doubt would disappear.

—Jennifer Michael Hecht, *Doubt: A History*

For as long as humans have understood it to be the wellspring
of thought, the brain has also evoked a singular curiosity, as
though it, unlike other parts of the body, could possess a life
force of its own. In ancient Greece, the brain was identified as the
origin point of thought around the fifth century BCE. In the late
fifteenth and early sixteenth centuries, Leonardo da Vinci searched
for the soul within the brain. Soon after, in sixteenth-century Italy,
brain dissections were theatrical events as well as educational ones—
Andreas Vesalius dissected brains in front of large audiences of
spectators and medical students, and his work was illustrated, in
woodcuts, in his book *The Fabric of the Human Body*. As understandings of the brain advanced, so, too, did questions about the origin points of illness and pain. It was in the seventeenth century that

anxiety came to be conceptualized as a condition having to do with problems of the nerves and, eventually, the brain.

To this day, scientists attempt to locate experiences and behaviors in the body and the brain. Research often asks questions like: Where is psychosis? Where is anxiety? Where is cancer, diabetes? Can they be found in our brains, and now, in our DNA? If we don't know the source of the problem, we struggle to treat it at its root. Anxiety, a state that is overwhelmingly physical in its presentation, pretends to lend itself to this sort of thinking—yet our understanding of it, and its treatment, can become constrained by this logic of geography. The story of anxiety and the body, and most of all, anxiety and the brain, is one of interaction: of the constant conversations that take place between our brains and other parts of our bodies, and between our brains and the world around us.

These days, when we think of anxiety, we think, first, of the brain. We think of our anxiety as the product of thoughts in particular—thoughts generated in our brains. Or we may think of anxiety as being due to too much activity in certain brain regions like the amygdala and the hippocampus, or due to the neurotransmitters at constant work within our brains, which have seemingly infinite potential for dysfunction. When we think in these concrete terms, it feels natural to place anxiety within the medical sphere, an illness that is contained entirely within the body just as much as, say, type 1 diabetes is, and one that could be explained in purely logical terms. And as much as this equation leaves me cold, there is comfort in it. If anxiety were fully explained by our bodily functions, there might be a cure at hand. But in fact, our brains are iterative organs, constantly adjusting to an ongoing dialogue with their biological and environmental surrounds. We are born with particular genetic predispositions that are later expressed, quieted, or even muted by our experiences—for better and for worse. These internal and external forces that shape our brains ultimately shape our lives.

An electrical, chemical entity governed, at least in part, by biological processes, the brain is also a symbol of reason and the centerpiece of emotional life. Though we've come to know far more about the inner workings of our brains that we did even a decade ago, they remain, in many respects, mysterious. The brain occupies a complicated place in the history of science and in modern thinking about health. To what degree are our brains rational, biological devices? And to what degree are they a place of passion, of spontaneity, outside the realm of data? We cling to the idea that our brains are swayed most powerfully by reason—more so than raw emotion, more so than inexplicable passions. We want them to guide us toward reasonable decisions, reasonable beliefs, and, most of all, reasonable feelings. Yet reason and feeling can be painfully at odds—even (especially) when we know better. Reason can be momentarily calming—yet unreasonable, unlikely, horrific, and also beautiful things happen every day. Things don't always work out. Even as I write these words, there's no denying that I am, in my way, trying to tame the chaos that surrounds us all. To understand anxiety and the brain requires an appreciation of data, yes, and feeling too.

When we experience anxiety, our feelings and our awareness of what is likely or true can fall out of sync. Attention can become consumed by fear. We wish for our brains to be mechanisms of sensemaking, as though if we could just be rational enough, life would be newly predictable and we could eradicate our uncertainties. We attempt to combat anxiety with logic, order, and distraction—by, say, thinking through the odds of one outcome or another, or by making lists of what we can and cannot change, or by watching mindless TV—often with little success. Most all of us are comforted by the concrete assurance of facts, but they are often a false promise. And though much of human experience is now subject to scientific inquiry, there is also a great deal that has to, simply, be felt.

In our brains, there are networks made up of different brain areas. Known as functional brain networks, these are systems that influence all aspects of our experience, from our emotional tendencies to our capacity to organize information or make plans. A recent meta-analysis on the differences in functional brain networks in people who do and do not struggle with anxiety found that in the brains of anxious people (with a wide variety of forms of anxiety), there was less connectivity in certain areas of the brain than in the nonanxious participants. In particular, they found lower levels of network connectivity among networks "responsible for the processing of perception, salience, and uncertainty." These reductions in connectivity suggest a breakdown in communication between the brain network that regulates emotion and the network that is associated with the organization and control of our thoughts. Intuitively, these findings make sense. When anxiety is high, affective (feeling) experience seems to override logic, order, and practical thought. Instead of the two working in harmony, they seem to miss each other.

Over the past century, the brain has often been compared to a computer. And although this comparison is generally made in an effort to better understand the incredibly complex inner workings of our minds, I find it tired and unsatisfying. For as much as our brains gather and evaluate information, they are also subject to the raw and often irrational forces of feeling, to our own idiosyncratic histories, and to the contexts in which we exist. Our anxieties, in all their complexity, force us to face the ways in which human experience resists oversimplification. After decades of conceptualizing brains as computers, it is no surprise that we are now being bombarded with claims that our brains and our anxieties can be "hacked." The promise of a quick fix is enticing. I've been tempted by all kinds of hacks for anxiety, from essential oils that will allegedly (if you buy them right! now!) eradicate anxiety at bedtime, to vitamins, to habit-tracking apps. Of course, attempts to employ shortcuts and oversimplifications to resolve complex problems lead to disappointment. Anxiety forces us to remember that we are not machines, and neither our brains nor our fears can be hacked.

State-of-the-art research on the human brain points toward its intricate, vast nature. Research on human connectomes, which are maps of our neural connections (sometimes compared to fingerprints), is beginning to expand our understanding of the ways in which anxiety manifests in terms of brain activity. The Human Connectome Project, which began in 2010, is attempting to construct a comprehensive map of the human brain—a truly monumental task. One arm of this work, known as the Human Connectome Project for Disordered Emotional States (HCP-DES) has taken up depression and anxiety in particular. They hope to be able to identify anxiety and depression not only on the basis of the symptoms that people describe but at the level of our brains' neural pathways. In a recent study looking at healthy individuals' brains, researchers were able to identify participants with anxiety symptoms on the basis of neural networks that impact emotion regulation, including the ventral attention network, which has implications for our capacity to shift our attention. The Human Connectome Project could, in time, have massive implications for the ways that we think about and treat anxiety. In part, work on the human connectome provides physical evidence of the ways that anxiety manifests in the brain. But even more so, I find that understanding the physiology of anxiety helps to illuminate the emotional experience of it, of how deeply entrenched it can be. The sense that reason, in and of itself, isn't enough or that the hacks don't work or that attention is not so easily moved—this bears out at the level of the brain.

In keeping with Western culture's current fixation on positivity, people often try to spin anxiety as entirely useful, as though we should be grateful for it. Contemporary thinking about anxiety emphasizes its evolutionary value—that anxiety is necessary—as it helps us to notice errors and, above all, avoid danger. Our brains work hard to keep us alive. In this sense, and even in its more modern permutations (there is, for instance, survival value in caring about whether you've left your stove on), there is no question that anxiety is necessary. And in earlier periods of human life, it was anxiety that kept us alert to predators—again, keeping us, quite literally, alive. It is essential that we notice threats in time to escape them. As babies, we need a degree of wariness of the unknown to prevent catastrophe. And across the lifespan, we need enough doubt, enough uncertainty, enough hesitation to exercise caution.

But with these old mechanics in place in our modern surroundings, anxiety emerges in circumstances in which it is no longer useful. Evolutionary value isn't much consolation when you feel bombarded by an outsize sense of risk at every turn. On their own, evolutionary explanations are inadequate. Anxiety is a response to internal states and external events that fall both within and outside the bounds of evolutionary explanations—but also, evolutionary explanations and existential concerns are fundamentally intertwined. Anxiety, this practical survival instinct generated by the body, is also a common symptom of existential crisis. Panic can feel, if briefly, like the end of the world. Survival instincts are about maintaining our existence, about going on—and so, too, are our existential fears. There is no escaping the limits of our lives, and most of all, no escaping our own mortality.

We know that a range of forms of anxiety can evoke analogous activity in the brain—but there appear to be important differences too. A recent meta-analysis looked at neurological responses to both induced anxiety (that is, anxiety deliberately evoked in a laboratory setting, often through electrical shocks at unpredictable intervals) and pathological anxiety (anxiety in the context of an anxiety disorder). Though researchers found a number of similarities, when they looked at the brain function of people with different *kinds* of anxiety disorders, they found that the brains of people with specific phobias—like, say, fear of heights or spiders or needles—appear more like the brains of people experiencing lab-induced anxiety than do the brains of people with other forms of anxiety, especially generalized anxiety disorder. We know that in the face of situations that obviously threaten our survival, we tap into that oldest form of anxiety, the anxiety that wants, most of all, to keep us alive. This anxiety may be neurologically akin to the anxiety that is kicked up for people with specific phobias—for a person who is afraid of heights, looking out the window of a skyscraper feels like a threat to their survival. Intuitively, this makes sense—the edge of a cliff presents an obvious danger. On the other hand, it may be that some forms of anxiety reflect struggles that aren't as clearly tied to basic survival instincts, as is often the case with chronic anxiety in conditions like GAD—and they may work differently at the level of the brain. It may be that there are some forms of anxiety that are closely tied to our evolutionary history, and other forms of anxiety that are warning us in different, new ways.

Beyond its evolutionary value, anxiety has another kind of utility hidden within it, one that strikes me as more timely and ultimately more useful, and one that doesn't require pretending to like it. Rather than attempting to fight anxiety solely with reason, or by trying to square the unsquarable, or with quick fixes that are doomed to fail, I've found far greater leverage in homing in on anxiety as a transitional process and a source of information. Anxiety can spur us on, it can insist that we find the way from one mental state to another. When, for instance, the sensations of anxiety emerge within our bodies, rather than attempting to push them away, we can begin to notice our emotional and environmental context. In this way, anxiety can point us toward previously obscured needs and wishes, and it can alert us to areas in which we yearn for change. Central to this process is attention—attention forms the bridge.

In the field of visual perception, there is a phenomenon known as inattentional blindness. Essentially, what you don't pay attention to, you literally don't see. Anxiety creates a similar sort of distortion in awareness—you experience only what you are paying attention to, and you lose out on a lot of good. The movement of our attention shapes our lives.

In a world in which you could fully control your attention, you probably wouldn't be very anxious, at least not consciously. Instead of reliving the details of an argument with a friend over and over, you might finish a task or make dinner. You might choose to attend to work or pleasure or any number of other things, but few would actively allot their hours to worry. But we do not live in that world, and our attention easily gets stuck. When we are anxious, our attention becomes fixed on whatever it is that feels threatening—even when there is nothing we can do about it, and even when what we perceive as a threat isn't, in reality, so threatening. And though there will never be a world free from worry, there can be one of greater freedom of thought. I think a lot about the ways we jostle our minds out of worry and fear, and how we live alongside our pain without so much struggle. Experience has shown me, time and time again, that berating oneself for worrying is counterproductive. This can contribute to low self-esteem and to depression, and as it turns the gaze inward, as anxiety tends to do, it absorbs attention.

When I think of the time that I have lost to anxiety—to uncertainties, to matters well outside the bounds of my influence—I am livid. I'll look back soon after a period of overwhelming worry, with the briefly held wisdom of hindsight, and wonder how else I could have spent my days had my attention been elsewhere. I am sickened by the thought of the periods of time in which my energy, and above all, my capacity for generative, creative thinking, have been overshadowed by fear and dread. I know that this anger needs to be put to some kind of use. Where might my attention land if it weren't consumed by anxiety? What might it be possible for me to experience, feel, do, instead? A sense of ownership over my own attention— that would be self-possession. So when I think about this time lost, I now think, too, about how else I might spend my time. The other side of rage can be potential.

Anxiety has a way of making even the most confident among us feel, albeit temporarily, fragile and raw. In myself and in my work, I've seen the many ways that anxiety wreaks havoc, even among people who are "high functioning," as we call it, people who are working, caring for families, and shouldering heavy responsibilities. It manifests visibly and invisibly, in the body and the mind, with symptoms ranging from muscle tension, headaches, and nausea, to avoidance, irritability, distraction, and inability to concentrate. The World Health Organization reports that the global economy loses about $1 trillion per year due to lost work deriving from depression and anxiety. This is a measurable, if cold (and, as measurable things often are, insufficient) proxy for the way anxiety sucks the air out of the proverbial room.

When we perceive a threat of any kind, our attention moves toward it. The spectrum of anxiety across which we all move is structured, in part, by our experiences of threat appraisal. We are all constantly evaluating our environments, even when we put little conscious effort into doing so (say, in the moment that we look both ways before crossing the street). Yet some of us appraise threats easily, without much friction, whereas others get stuck in the threat-appraisal process or feel threat where it isn't. Threat perception shapes your experiences of what threat *feels* like. For some people, for whom anxiety isn't a constant, a bit of threat can feel more like an adventure, like something to conquer. For others, it feels like total destruction on the horizon—perpetual and exhausting.

Anxiety flourishes and expands in small and large moments of interpretation—moments that we all face frequently, whether we're aware of it or not. Will I go ahead and eat the yogurt that expires today? Cross the street with ten seconds remaining before the light changes? Get an epidural? Is this a moment of high or moderate risk? Is this a chance worth taking? Or: How precarious will I allow my body to be today (as though I really have a choice)? What strikes me as a worrisome sensation or a reckless behavior might to most others be a neutral or even thrilling experience (I've found myself across the street from my husband at a stoplight, waiting for what I see as a slightly safer moment to cross, many times). The balance between risk and reward becomes skewed, with concerns about risk taking up so much space that they push other interests and experiences out of mind entirely.

Put in practical terms: You may want to be attending to, thinking about, feeling immersed in a conversation with a friend, or playing with your child, or reading a book. But attention often wanders to worries—like the well-being of loved ones or a problem at work. Attention is easily consumed by these perceived threats, stuck there, far away from things that bring about joy and fulfillment. Most of us have experienced this pull away from the life in front of us, yet it is difficult to shift. And this is borne out in research—threat is processed differently by people who are prone to anxiety. A seminal meta-analysis on anxiety and threat perception found that across age groups and anxiety disorders, people who are anxious pay more attention to threat than people who aren't anxious. Another meta-analysis found that even when looking through the lens of brain activity, people who experience anxiety "allocate more attentional resources toward disorder-congruent negative stimuli," meaning that when an anxious person's particular alarm bells are activated—perhaps the car in front of them brakes suddenly, or they feel a sharp pain in their back—they direct more attention toward what is concerning them than nonanxious people do. Anxiety does not resolve solely by seeing the error in one's thinking or by exercising reasonable thought. One can understand, on an intellectual level, that a situation is not particularly threatening, that your anxiety is unfounded—yet feel, nonetheless, overwhelmed by a sense of looming catastrophe.

Anxiety is especially disruptive when attention becomes stuck in one place or another, seemingly immovable. I treated a woman in her thirties who was, by all accounts, extraordinarily successful. She had recently made partner at a large law firm and was mother to a young child. She described a happy marriage and a fulfilling social life. But when her father was diagnosed with a serious but treatable illness, she became consumed with worry about his prognosis. She would spend long hours researching the treatment options available to him but struggled to focus on work or on her home life. She described feeling constantly distracted, as though her thoughts about her father's illness and treatment had taken up all the space in her mind—that is, her attention was utterly consumed. She soon developed debilitating panic attacks that would interrupt her workday two to three times a week. First, she would notice that her hands were shaking and her heart was racing and then she would begin to sweat profusely and feel as though she were going to vomit or faint. She would rush out of her office, terrified that she was going to be humiliated in front of her colleagues or that she was going to die of a heart attack at her desk and leave her child without a mother. This kind of derailment of attention is far more harmful than fewer items checked off a list—it becomes a form of suffering.

Research on anxiety and the brain has for some time emphasized the amygdala, a small region located in both hemispheres of the brain, and its role in responding to threat. And there is no doubt that the amygdala is one of the primary hubs of fear in the brain. But researchers are also now highlighting the importance of another area in the brain called the bed nucleus of the stria terminalis (BNST) and its importance in making sense of anxiety disorders at a neurological level. The BNST may be particularly important for the experience of hypervigilance—a state in which we are on high alert for threats—whereas the amygdala may be more involved when we face imminent danger. In more human terms, this distinction is useful in understanding the varying experiences of, on one hand, constantly scanning a room or a street for potential harm, even in the absence of any evident threat, or, on the other hand, noticing that someone is, in fact, running toward you with a knife. Hypervigilance—that constant state of looking out for possible threats—consumes a great deal of attention.

There is also some evidence of structural differences in the brains of people with anxiety—for instance, that in the brains of people with generalized anxiety disorder, there seems to be less gray matter in certain areas than in the brains of people without evidence of any mental illness. In particular, researchers have found that for people with GAD, some of the areas of the brain that are linked to attention are actually smaller than those in the brains of people without GAD, and they explain that these structural differences may have to do with "attentional deficits linked to excessive worry." So, for people with GAD, it may be that brain structures and their function play a central role in how difficult it can be to extricate oneself from worry. To move away from worry requires attentional control.

We can think about attention and anxiety at the level of the brain and in social contexts too. A study conducted in the Netherlands looked at the ways in which anxiety and attention work within families, and how anxiety is transmitted among family members. The study was conducted over the course of two points in time, first when children were 4.5 years old and then when they were 7.5 years old. Researchers found that among parents who were higher in anxiety at the first assessment, their children demonstrated attentional bias to threat at the second assessment. That is, over time, the children of anxious parents seemed to develop heightened attention for threat—and we know that heightened attention for threat is linked to anxiety. It is easy to imagine the scenarios in which this unfolds, despite our best intentions. A parent with anxious proclivities may inadvertently emphasize and, in turn, model, high awareness of threats in the world in an effort to keep their child out of harm's way. And children have a way of noticing our every move.

I spoke to Alexander Shackman, PhD, an expert on the biology of anxiety and a faculty member at the University of Maryland. I'm interested in the ways that Shackman's work on neuroimaging (for instance, MRI technology) and anxiety can help us to understand the ways that attentional bias to threat play out in the context of anxiety. We talked about how anxiety is associated with an inflexibility of attention, and he explained that "individuals who have a tougher time flexibly allocating their attention and regulating their thoughts are more likely to develop anxiety disorders." In keeping with Shackman's description, research shows that attention is a central aspect of emotion regulation, though we don't always talk about it in those terms, and that having a degree of control over one's attention may help to mitigate problems tolerating difficult emotional states. The ability that each of us has to regulate our thoughts and emotions, or the degree to which we struggle to do so, is central to our well-being. Attention and emotion are powerfully intertwined aspects of our functioning. They shape our subjective experience of our day-to-day lives. Without the ability to shift attention, we lose the ability to regulate our thoughts and emotions. As I spoke to Shackman, I reflected on having seen this phenomenon of inflexible attention and anxiety play out in my clinical experience, and also, that it feels, intuitively, on point. And as our conversation unfolded, I realized what it is that I've been circling around all this time, what I've struggled with myself and seen in patients. What I want to know most of all is: Can we think about anxiety as a problem of attention? Shackman said, "I think we can."

Yes. Anxiety is a problem of attention.

When we are anxious, our attention (and, as a consequence, our time and energy) tends to be diverted inward. Focus moves toward internal experiences, like, say, an ache in the back, or yesterday's difficult conversation at work. This inward movement is an effort to find safety—in that it can feel like a way to prevent disaster, or to find a shred of reassurance that disaster isn't looming. But it is also a trap. It can lead to isolation, and it tends to be circular. Little room is left for engaging with the world outside, without which it becomes difficult to move forward in one's mind. But by effortfully noticing the movement of our attention and where it seems to become stuck, we can start to learn about the ways that our anxiety moves our minds.

Our attention is finite, and its direction dictates much of our emotional lives. Imagine peering inside the mind of a so-called workaholic, someone whose energy, time, and above all, attention, is centered on work. Inevitably, this comes at the expense of other areas of their life. Work is the focal point of their attention, and as a result, other parts of life—time with family and friends, or a hobby, aren't. This person might receive professional accolades and promotions, and yet feel a nagging sense of loneliness. Then, imagine a person who develops an intense passion for running. They go to work, they see their friends and family, but what they think about in their spare time, and the way that they spend much of their early mornings and weekends, is training for races. Their diet is shaped around running. Over lunch and before bed, they watch YouTube videos on optimal training. And now, imagine a person with chronic, significant anxiety. You go to work, you care for your family. But in spare moments, instead of finding space for curiosity or relaxation, your attention is sunk into a kind of black hole of worry, whether about work or family or health or any number of other matters. These are very different minds to occupy, and very different lives to live. To understand anxiety, and to treat it effectively, we have to attend to our attention— where it is, and where we want it to be.

We know that the movement of our attention dictates much of our lives, and that it influences the ways we interact with the world and the ways we experience ourselves. Yet we often feel as though we have little, if any, control over it. Our attention is drawn one way or another, or we become entirely engrossed, or we feel as though we can't pay attention at all, even to things of importance to us. We struggle with the places our minds are drawn to. In psychotherapy, as both a patient and as a therapist, you become acutely aware of what you and other people attend to—what do we see? And even more so, what do we miss? What strikes us as interesting, and what do we move past without much thought? Although our attention is finite, it can also be flexible.

The importance of attention and its movement has been at the heart of philosophical and religious practices for thousands of years, as in Buddhist teachings. Today, secular mindfulness practices tend to emphasize the ways in which we can learn to modulate our own attention, with an eye toward remaining in the present moment, rather than drifting into the past or the future. In the now classic book on mindfulness and well-being, *Full Catastrophe Living*, Jon Kabat-Zinn, PhD, a professor of medicine and prolific writer and teacher, explains: "Mindfulness is cultivated by paying close attention to your moment-to-moment experience while, as best you can, not getting caught up in your ideas and opinions, likes and dislikes." Kabat-Zinn is the founder of mindfulness-based stress reduction (MBSR), a practice that integrates meditation and yoga. And though MBSR was initially developed in a hospital setting, Kabat-Zinn saw it, too, as a "public health intervention." Indeed, its reach has since extended from the sphere of health care into other settings like schools and prisons. It is used around the world and across the lifespan, with children as well as with the elderly. MBSR has been found to be useful in managing a range of conditions, from chronic pain to high blood pressure to asthma, and it is consistently associated with a reduction in symptoms of anxiety. A recent study even found that MBSR was as effective as escitalopram (an antidepressant that is often used to treat anxiety disorders) in reducing anxiety symptoms. We see, over and over, that our attention and our well-being are intimately intertwined.

The question of how to shift one's mind, especially during hard times, is also at the heart of psychotherapy. How do we work through our distress while also moving forward? Some forms of treatment focus on containing anxiety. For instance, cognitive therapists sometimes ask patients to schedule "worry time," which is time in which you devote your attention solely to, well, worrying. According to this method, any time your attention is drawn toward worries outside the specified worry window, you should attempt to redirect it and essentially save the worry for later. Other treatment methods focus on mindfulness techniques and are geared toward observing and acknowledging when your attention is drawn toward a worry and developing tolerance for the distress associated with it. Yet other treatment methods are interested in understanding the places anxiety seems to draw our attention to, with the idea being that through insight and understanding, we can find greater freedom in our minds.

Understanding the role of attention in anxiety and developing a degree of attentional control is not synonymous with avoidance or repression. When attention feels unwieldy, the goal is not to sweep worries under the rug through constant distraction—from there, they will most certainly return. Instead, with practice, we get to know the particular permutations of our anxieties and of our minds. Maybe one day we can say, "Oh that? That is my anxiety at work. I see it, I know it well. I won't ignore it, yet I also won't be held hostage by it."

It is often said that we should pay attention to what our minds are "marinating in," because we take on the essence of that which surrounds us. And in fact, our brains are constantly swimming through our surrounds, internal, social, and environmental. Despite the chaos that we are all, inevitably, immersed in, we can learn to build rich inner worlds populated by the things that fascinate us, that excite us—that is, the things that we want to direct our attention to. In this way, we can protect ourselves from some of anxiety's reach. This is a modern survival instinct, and it is the opposite of a hack.

We are capable of many kinds of attention, some of which even work in opposition to anxiety. Just as mindfulness practices can help us to attend to the present moment, we can also cultivate the ability to allow our minds to shift, thoughtfully, from one place to another. We need to have periods of unstructured thought in which our minds can meander and draw connections. I'm thinking of a state that hovers somewhere between reverie, diffuse thinking, and digression, all of which share a fluidity from which unexpected connections can emerge. "Reverie," a term used in psychoanalytic circles, is akin to daydreaming, and diffuse thinking is a related concept. Barbara Oakley, PhD, an engineer who writes about learning and the brain, explains, "Diffuse-mode thinking is what happens when you relax your attention and just let your mind wander." Digression takes many forms—sometimes it happens in a conversation that moves from place to place organically, or in a chain of thought that emerges and takes a shape that you didn't anticipate. When you allow yourself to float between thoughts, you cultivate flexible attention—rather than remaining stuck in a repetitive, at times agonizing, cycle of worry and accompanying frustration. Often, we realize that we've been in these open, even creative states of mind after the fact—when, for instance, a solution to a problem at work that you've been wrestling with for days occurs to you while you are cleaning or taking a walk, instead of when you sit down to focus directly on the issue. Or when we fantasize about the future or feel the rush of potential nearing.

In the mid-1970s, psychologist Mihaly Csikszentmihalyi coined the now famous term "flow," and thus began a field of research on this elusive yet important and even pleasurable state of mind. More recently, flow has been characterized as "a state of total absorption in an activity, involving focused attention, deep engagement, loss of self-conscious awareness, and self-perceived temporal distortion." I spoke to Cameron Norsworthy, PhD, a scientist and coach who studies the science of flow, about the relationship between anxiety and flow states. Flow is often linked to extreme sports—for instance, the state of mind of a rock climber at their best (and there's also a considerable body of work on the role of flow for musicians). Norsworthy has a long history as an athlete himself, and now he trains professional athletes and is the CEO of the Flow Centre. We talked about the ways that flow extends into all sorts of contexts—not only athletics. One could experience flow while writing, for instance, or even during quotidian tasks like washing the dishes. Flow is a state of mind, a kind of attention, that most of us strive for—we might get good work done during flow, and also, it feels good. Flow can even be a buffer for daily stress. And here's the part that I'm most fascinated by: flow and anxiety are *mutually exclusive*—they cannot co-occur.

When we sit down to work, or at the piano, or when we go out for a run, we don't enter into a flow state immediately. Rather, as I heard it described by flow expert Josh Dickson, flow seems to unfold within a cycle, a cycle that begins with "struggle." Dickson explains that the period of struggle before entering a flow state may be characterized by anxiety or by trouble focusing one's attention—but "flow cannot be cheated." It is only through tolerating the discomfort, the anxiety that precedes flow, that you open the door to it.

Sometimes, flow happens in surprising ways. When I look back at that period of anxiety and depression in my late twenties, I think of embroidery. For a time, embroidery became, for me, an unexpected haven. A truly ancient art form, there is evidence of embroidery dating back thousands of years (from, for instance, ancient Egypt and ancient China). Embroidery has always had a particular power, one that is built on the intertwining of beauty and necessity, from its use in documenting historical events to communicating wishes and beliefs, making declarations of identity, and even summoning protection. I started with sashiko, a Japanese form of embroidery, one that I chose on the basis of its apparent simplicity. I later learned that sashiko is, in fact, intricate and complex. It originated as a reparative art—historically, it was used to strengthen garments and extend their lives. It requires precision and patience and attention. Then, emboldened, I embroidered a mermaid with 3D metallic hair. Soon after, it was Christmas gnomes riding mice. And in the months that followed, when I became pregnant, I embroidered real and imaginary animals on linen—dragons, wolves, crabs, squirrels, more mermaids. Little by little, I started to notice the return of a creative, generative kind of attention that had previously been obscured by worry and dread, a state in which my thoughts were gentle and focused, and new ideas began to emerge. In these newfound moments of flow, embroidery became a way for me to reengage with my own lush interiority and to repopulate myself with vitality instead of dread.

For as much as we've learned about the brain, we have only just begun. A recent study—a massive one—found only negligible differences in the brain structures of people with generalized anxiety when compared to healthy controls. Another study is now calling into question the findings of many brain-wide association studies (BWAS), which have been at the center of a great deal of research in recent years. These studies use magnetic resonance imaging (MRIs) to look at differences in brain anatomy and function in order to identify relationships between these differences and experiences of mental illness or other forms of disease. BWAS bring with them the hope of shedding light on the neurological underpinnings of so many of our ailments. But despite so much promise, these new findings suggest that many studies of this kind did not include enough participants to provide solid, dependable results—and that they will actually need to include a minimum of thousands of participants, casting doubt on years of research. In the immense complexity of the brain, we see that things change. The state of the art evolves. The work is ongoing, always reshaping itself.

Soma, in Latin, means body. And the soma is the body of a neuron, home to many of its essential functions. The brain is made up of some eighty-six billion neurons, whose dynamic activities and communication are at the center of our well-being. With this tiny yet elemental component of mental life, we are reminded of the body in the brain and the brain in the body. In the utter vastness of the brain, so much can go wrong, and so much can go right—and we are only just beginning to understand. What do we have to hold on to, how do we steady ourselves? It turns out, what we do have, for sure, is our attention. To appreciate its movement, and to exercise a degree of authority within one's own mind—this is real power in the face of anxiety, self-possession of the highest kind.

CURIOSITY AND FLEXIBILITY

How big a piece of "reality" can man bite off
without narrowing it down distortingly?

—Ernest Becker, *The Denial of Death*

A nxiety, by all of its many names, is characterized by feeling
stuck—fixed in places we wish we weren't. This feeling of
stuckness can manifest as thoughts or worries, or as compulsive behaviors, or in our relationships. Often, it is precisely this sense
of not knowing how to do *something else* that drives people to finally
pursue therapy. Why is it that we find ourselves stuck in patterns of
feeling and behavior? Why do certain thoughts seem to follow us no
matter how we attempt to dismiss them? Anxiety can be the product
of a sort of neurological path of least resistance, with our brains becoming accustomed to the patterns of neural activity that accompany
it. As the oft-quoted saying goes, "Neurons that fire together wire

together." We are pulled toward repetition rather than change. This is a matter of our physiology, and of our psychology too.

We have all, will all, sometimes feel stuck in thoughts or behaviors that trouble us—it is part of being alive. When it comes to more significant, chronic anxiety, these periods of feeling stuck can become consuming—of time, of energy, of attention. Unwanted, unbidden worries and their sequelae assert themselves, and uncertainty becomes increasingly hard to bear. This happens in the context of generalized anxiety disorder, for instance—and also, it is central to obsessive-compulsive disorder. OCD is, for the person experiencing it, insistent, unbending, an anxiety that is perpetual, at once boring and infernal. When it comes to feeling, to put it mildly, stuck, OCD is the ultimate teacher.

OCD is thought to have to do, at least in part, with overactivity in a network of interconnected parts of the brain known as the cortico-striato-thalamo-cortical (CSTC) loop. The CSTC loop impacts, among other things, repetitive behaviors—and its overactivity is thought to contribute to the experience of feeling locked in a repetitive cycle. OCD is defined, primarily, by frequent obsessions and/or compulsions, and most people diagnosed with OCD experience both. Obsessions are painful for the person experiencing them. They can manifest as thoughts, images, or impulses—and they evoke feelings of dread, disgust, horror, and despair: "I see a drop of water on the floor. If I don't clean it up completely, someone could slip on it and die, and it will be my fault" or "What if I involuntarily drive my car off this bridge?" or "What if I throw my dog out the window by accident?" or "What if the salad I made for a dinner party was contaminated with salmonella and all of my guests die as a result?"

Obsessive thinking is perseverative—that is, it persists, against one's will, it feels unshakable. It is for this reason that the word "sticky" is often used to describe patterns of thinking in OCD.

Like obsessions, compulsions can take many forms, from cleaning to checking to asking for reassurance. Compulsions are, in essence, an attempt to counteract obsessions. When we are obsessive, we become consumed with thoughts that disturb us. And when we are compulsive, our attempts to neutralize these thoughts with our actions are generally irrational, even to the person thinking, feeling, and doing them. One might think, for instance, "If I line my shoes up neatly in my closet, no harm will come to my family" or "If I tap each of the dials on the stove three times after checking that they are off, my daughter won't die in a fire." That these links are irrational is usually well known to the person making them, yet not a powerful enough feeling to stop the cycle. But compulsions are more than an irrational attempt to prevent disaster. By lining up our shoes or checking the stove, what we are really after is an elusive (impossible) sense of certainty.

Just as anxiety exists on a continuum, so, too, do obsessions and compulsions. You can have inclinations, or you can have a full-blown disorder. In fact, obsessive and compulsive tendencies are quite common, even among people who do not meet criteria for OCD. Most of us are inclined to think obsessively and to act compulsively when we are particularly anxious. And like anxiety, in small doses obsessions and compulsions can have their advantages. People prone to a bit of obsessionality and compulsivity are often praised at work or school because they notice problems before they've unfolded, and in so doing, they may occasionally succeed in preventing them. Even within the diagnostic spectrum, mild forms of OCD can be frustrating and distressing at times, but they don't interfere in any extreme sense with one's life. But as you continue along the spectrum of obsessionality and compulsivity, rather than preventing problems, they emerge needlessly. OCD can be severe, and for some people, it can be a constant, all-consuming, lifelong struggle.

OCD tends to overlap with other anxiety disorders and mood disorders (e.g., depression) rather than existing in isolation. A recent meta-analysis found that in a sample of fifteen thousand people with a diagnosis of OCD, two thirds of them also had another psychiatric diagnosis. In the same study, among children diagnosed with OCD, the most common comorbid diagnosis (meaning that a person is diagnosed with both conditions) was an anxiety disorder, whereas in adults diagnosed with OCD, the most common comorbid diagnosis was a mood disorder. The researchers who conducted this study point out that it could be the case that the fallout of OCD symptoms over the course of life could contribute to problems with mood in adulthood. It may be that over time, OCD symptoms are, basically, exhausting, and if they are untreated, eventually, depression comes around too.

The DSM is updated periodically, and in its most recent iteration, OCD was moved out of the category of anxiety disorders and into a new category called obsessive-compulsive and related disorders (OCRDs). This category includes diagnoses like trichotillomania (compulsive hair-pulling, for instance, pulling out one's eyelashes), and excoriation disorder (compulsive skin picking). The argument to create this new category of diagnoses is based in large part on the fact that these conditions involve repetitive behaviors—whether cleaning or hair pulling or skin picking, to name a few. This marks a controversial shift, and it is one that some OCD experts have taken issue with. From a clinical perspective, I take issue with this recategorization. I continue to think of OCD under the same umbrella as I do anxiety disorders, and I believe that a discussion of anxiety disorders is incomplete without also addressing OCD. You would be hardpressed to find a person with OCD who doesn't feel anxious.

Jonathan Abramowitz, PhD, is a psychologist at the University of North Carolina at Chapel Hill and one of the foremost experts on OCD and anxiety disorders in the United States. Abramowitz, along with psychologist Ryan Jacoby, have methodically articulated the reasons for which moving OCD out of the anxiety disorders category is problematic. At the heart of their argument, they point to the anxiety, that is, the sense of threat, that underlies OCD. When I spoke to Abramowitz about his critique of the recategorization of OCD in the DSM-5, his expertise in both the research and clinical spheres came through immediately—he spoke about OCD with sensitivity and depth. We talked about the ways in which it seems that anxiety simply cannot be untangled from OCD. And during our conversation, he introduced me to a term that I can't forget: "tender conscience." Applied to obsessions in a modern context by psychologist Stanley Rachman, whose pioneering work delved deeply into the human subtleties of OCD and anxiety more broadly, the term "tender conscience" gets at the pernicious nature of obsessive thinking, and at the internal, at times torturous experience of OCD itself. Rachman refers to the work of William James: "He argued that when people 'of tender conscience and religiously quickened' become unhappy, they experience 'moral remorse and compunction of feeling inwardly vile and wrong.'" *Inwardly vile and wrong.*

I read the term "tender conscience" as a kind one, borne out of empathy and curiosity. Now, when I think about what it means to live with a tender conscience, whether in the context of anxiety or OCD, I think of feeling the weight of decisions and outcomes heavily, of considering and reconsidering, and of feeling vast responsibility. I think of seeing around the bend, too far, too soon, of craving certainty, and above all, of feeling bound. How could this not redound to anxiety?

Perseverative thoughts, which is to say, those thoughts you feel stuck in, are a hallmark of anxiety. This sort of thinking can happen to all of us ("I'm going to fail my economics exam" or "I'll never find an apartment" on repeat), but they are especially present in obsessive-compulsive disorder, and in extremes, they can contribute to depressive symptoms. Perseverative thinking, for the person stuck in it, can feel like a (torturesome) attempt to resolve a problem, in which flexibility feels impossible. One might turn a past or upcoming event over and over in one's mind, as though with enough thought, a regrettable moment or a feared outcome could take on new meaning— as though every potential disaster could be anticipated, and thus prevented, every hint at a wrong righted. One might, then, be said to have a tender conscience.

Perseverative thinking, whether in the context of OCD or anxiety more broadly, can become a self-fulfilling prophecy. I recall a patient who had come to treatment struggling with constant worry that left him distracted and often unable to enjoy his children, his friends, or his minimal free time. He worried over his decisions unendingly, and he anticipated outcomes far beyond what he could possibly control. He explained to me, triumphant, that after having struggled with a days-old conversation with his boss that had left him distraught, after he'd turned it over and over in his mind ad nauseum, trying to find a way to perceive it that would allow him to settle himself, a small detail emerged—something he'd previously forgotten—and having recalled this minor detail, he felt newly at ease. He explained to me that his perseveration had worked. It had, eventually, brought on a sense of resolution. In this way, perseverative thinking can reinforce itself. We tend to recall the few occasions in which it leads somewhere that relieves our anxiety, and to disregard the reality that in the balance, perseveration and obsessive thinking broadly cause far more pain than they prevent. They consume time and energy better placed elsewhere, and they pull us inward, away from our lives.

But what is it that makes this perseverative sort of thought so powerful? Why are some of us, despite our own good judgment, pulled into this cycle? Research suggests that the five components that underlie perseverative thinking are "cognitive dyscontrol, self-focus, interpersonal content, valence, and uncertainty." As one who has been both subject and witness to a great deal of perseverative thinking and its inevitable consequences, these findings give shape to the particular pain that this sort of thinking can bring about. Rather than a mass of nonspecific, unrelenting anxiety, we see the threads that consistently run through perseverative thought. And though we are all subject to our own idiosyncratic constellations of experience, little imagination is required to see that feeling some combination of being out of control of one's thoughts, internally focused, concerned with relationship dynamics, and riddled with negative emotion and doubt is surely a kind of suffering.

A thought occurs to you, seemingly out of nowhere, and then you can't seem to escape it. It could be: Is this slight asymmetry in my musculature an indication of an underlying degenerative disease? Or, back to the realm of what is likely: Is it simply a product of the normal asymmetries of the human body? After all, you have never noticed it before, nor has it ever caused you any problems. But then: If you follow reason, if you ignore this, if you are so bold as to move forward with your day, you could miss the chance to pursue what could be lifesaving treatment. The regret could be all-consuming.

This is an impossible bind.

What is it that we need when we feel stuck in an anxious tailspin, what is it that is missing? Often, it is a kind of internal flexibility. Just as a degree of flexibility in our musculature is critical for our bodily health, so, too, are cognitive and emotional flexibility necessary for our mental health. Cognitive flexibility and emotional flexibility are, broadly speaking, what they sound like. Cognitive flexibility allows us to move from one task to another, and to move our attention accordingly, and emotional flexibility refers to our ability to shift our emotional responses. Research consistently shows that anxiety is associated with reduced cognitive flexibility. A recent study compared cognitive flexibility in people with generalized anxiety disorder, obsessive compulsive disorder, and healthy controls. They found that people with GAD and OCD were less cognitively flexible than healthy controls, and that those with OCD had even lower levels of cognitive flexibility than those with GAD. Another study found that emotional rigidity got in the way of the improvement of anxiety symptoms. The consequences of a lack of flexibility manifest broadly—from trouble with decision-making and problem-solving to reduced creativity.

Alongside cognitive flexibility, a related concept, emotional regulation, factors into how we cope with painful feelings or periods in our lives. Emotion regulation refers to the ways in which we are able to modulate and shift our emotional states. It is "the processes by which individuals influence which emotions they have, when they have them, and how they experience and express these emotions." Research suggests that lower levels of resilience are associated with higher levels of anxiety and depression, and that emotion regulation plays a role in this relationship.

The lucky among us, some of whom are circumstantially and dispositionally advantaged in this regard, learn effective emotion regulation at a young age. They may feel in their own skin much of the time, comfortable in their bodies. They seem to know, naturally, how to create equilibrium for themselves. To watch a certain movie, to make a comforting meal, to call a friend. It's knowledge they carry with them without too much searching. But then, for many people, emotion regulation is effortful, even in adulthood. Rather than having an internal sense of how to relate to and shift a difficult state of mind, of how to find equilibrium, it requires learning and practicing. And as essential as emotion regulation is, it isn't often taught. For this reason, it can become a fundamental goal of psychotherapy, one with potential for a great deal of growth.

The word "regulation" leaves a lot to be desired—as though we are computers or thermostats. But the principles that underpin emotion regulation aren't about numbing out, nor are they about arriving at a constant state of unflappability. Instead, emotion regulation is about developing a capacity for measured response and for a kind of bounce, for flexibility. We want to be capable of calm, of serenity, and we also want to be capable of wild joy, of outrage, of sadness, grief—this full spectrum of human feeling—without fearing that we will not be able to return from the depths. This capacity to emotionally regulate oneself, whether in the face of uncomfortable thoughts or feelings or circumstances, is essential to resilience.

Obsessive thinking gets in the way of cognitive and emotional flexibility and emotional regulation. It does not restrict itself to the brain—rather, it roams throughout the body. The anxiety creeps in, until eventually it takes over. There is the thought and then there is the thought's sequelae. A loss of appetite. A stress headache. The heart rate increases. Muscles tense. Soon, the fog of false urgency sets in. And this urgency can contribute to behaving impulsively—from impulsively asking for reassurance to impulsively researching medical concerns online to impulsively drinking. The impulsivity we experience in these moments grows out of the wish to get rid of the anxiety as quickly as possible. As anxiety rises, so, too, does impulsivity (and, conversely, when the anxiety burns off, so does the impulsivity). And this experience bears out in research: people with symptoms of anxiety have, in some studies, been found to have higher levels of impulsivity than people without anxiety.

Impulsivity is often a rigid, inflexible way of reacting to the discomfort in our lives. Maybe you respond to anxiety by immediately seeking reassurance, or by avoiding hard conversations altogether, or by drinking. With so little room between the anxiety and the reaction that follows, things repeat themselves, and new ways of being fail to emerge. Through this lens, learning to work through anxiety can become a kind of damage control. When you begin to notice the urgency and impulsivity that anxiety can evoke and then to proceed instead with care, with curiosity, you may actually avoid making decisions you wish you hadn't.

ᘓ

Anxiety is often dismissed as irrationality, or if not dismissed, framed as a failure in thinking, a failure of the brain. But is anxiety really a failure of reason? On the one hand, yes, anxiety does often hover over unlikely outcomes and improbable catastrophes. But on the other hand, it is also true that we have very little control over the strokes of luck or twists of fate that dictate our lives, and that, quite frankly, is terrifying. To my mind, this is the central paradox of anxiety—it is at once entirely unreasonable and profoundly logical. It's not that I think disaster is the most likely outcome, but that I can't entirely rule it out. Glorious surprises and horrific tragedies happen. But even if you accept that the mess and unruliness of life is inescapable, somewhere along the line, anxiety drifts further away from reason, as it distorts probabilities and likelihoods. And reason also stops being a useful metric. We believe a lot of unreasonable things. Consider a common superstition like knocking on wood. You probably don't believe that saying "knock on wood" (or even actually doing it) will offer any true protection, but an awful lot of us do it *just in case.* Our anxieties are not cured with logic and lists, probabilities, and good sense alone.

We look for power, however elusive, in all kinds of ways. And sometimes our methods are in blatant opposition to our own logically held, reasonable beliefs. We all have a tendency to imbue thoughts, actions, and even words with false meaning, and in so doing, to determine relationships among things. This is known as magical thinking, or, as it manifests in other contexts, superstition. Magical thinking is part of everyday life, even in the absence of clinical anxiety. Stuart Vyse, a psychologist who studies superstition, writes, "If there is a universal truth about superstition, it is that superstitious behavior emerges as a response to uncertainty—to circumstances that are inherently random and uncontrollable." And it shows us that even for people who consider themselves logical, practical thinkers, sometimes our emotional needs can override practical thoughts and behaviors. When sports fans are compelled to wear particular socks on game day, this is magical thinking. When we knock on wood or cross our fingers, this, too, is magical thinking. And we can look to language, too, as in, for instance, the tendency to follow up a nasty comment about someone who has died with "God rest her soul." In this small way, we attempt to absolve ourselves of a bit of guilt or undo our regrets, that nastiness that we fear within ourselves. And we ask: With my thoughts, can I make things happen, or, can I stop things from falling apart? With my words, can I soothe my fears, my worries, my despair?

Magical thinking is a common feature of anxiety disorders, and of OCD too. If we imbue the action of, say, lining up our shoes in a particular order with the power to prevent a plane crash, despite the fact that we know this is not possible, it's a temporary comfort to quiet the terrifying awareness that our loved one on that plane could, will, eventually, die, at some unforeseeable time. You close the kitchen drawer fully—no harm will come to your child. Which is followed by the thought, "That's absurd, that isn't how things work," which is followed by the thought, "I'll do it, just in case." And therein lies the point—though it is obvious that none of these actions makes any difference, that they have nothing whatsoever to do with the well-being of one's family—we sometimes do them *just in case.* In this way, magical thinking is a portal into anxiety and OCD in particular. For a moment, we feel a little bit calmer—yet the relief is fleeting. Inevitably, something else comes up. With anxiety, if it's not one thing, it's only a matter of time before it's another.

But then, when we look closely, we find that magical thinking does have a certain power: it shows us our fears. And we see that just as we try to anchor ourselves in a sense of control—that, for instance, *a* causes *b,* however absurd (that the fully closed drawer will ensure safety), paradoxically, on the other side, what we tend to find is that it is the prospect of too much control that is most terrifying.

So, how powerful am I? It can be a comfort to remember that the answer, for nearly all of us, is: not very.

I'm buying crystals in Los Angeles. I've gone out of my way to do this, put time aside to travel to a neighborhood far from where I'm staying. It's been a difficult few months, and I'm feeling on edge. Anxiety has a way of doing this, temporarily stripping away one's confidence. So I've gone to buy crystals with a friend who really believes in them. A few nights before, sitting at dinner, she pulls upward of five pounds of crystals out of the pockets of her jacket. To me, this idea that crystals will quell my anxiety is, on the surface, absurd. I'm a psychologist, a scientifically minded person—and I'm skeptical by nature. But I suppose that even so, a part of me wants to believe, and in this fragile state of mind, I'm willing to try most anything. A crystal could be something to, quite literally, hold on to. If I carry this stone with me, if I stash it in my desk, maybe I could be stronger, more powerful. Maybe, somehow, since reason fails so often, this will protect me.

Or maybe the crystals could work because, with that tiny seed of belief within me, which doesn't really have anything to do with the crystals themselves, I could find my way to that emotional bridge that takes me from how I'm feeling now to a stronger, more courageous state—a state of flexibility instead of stuckness, one that I'm struggling to access but which I can feel nonetheless, dormant within me.

Years later, I'm in a coffee shop that sells evil-eye key chains at the register. I impulsively buy one for my husband. To protect him. Did I do this on an especially trying day? Maybe. Being reasonable, of course I don't believe this key chain has any capacity whatsoever to protect him. Somehow, though, buying it feels worthwhile. In these moments, I feel my sense of cause and effect and my emotional drive to protect, to prevent disaster and loss, pulling at each other.

It is often said that when you are anxious, it can be helpful to consider whether the thing on your mind will matter in the future, and then, whether you have any control over its outcome. Will this concern matter to me in a week, in a year? Will this matter to me when I'm ninety-five years old? Do any steps exist for me to influence its outcome? And for some forms of anxiety, this is helpful. These tend to be worries like: Is so-and-so mad at me? (You could have an honest conversation with them.) Or did I speak poorly in that meeting? (You could prepare more thoroughly next time.) But when anxiety is centered around more profound concerns like loss, death, and their sequelae, over which we have little, if any, control, it dissipates only when you zoom out beyond your own lifetime. Will my health matter in a hundred years? No. Even in the best of cases, in a hundred years I'll be dead. But in my lifetime, and within the scope of my small circle, my health matters enormously. It dictates the length of my time with my family. When anxiety is tied up in fears of loss and death, it isn't easily shaken off.

Although there is no doubt in my mind that anxiety is partially a matter of control, I bristle at the thought. The link between anxiety and control rings trite, clichéd, even square. It points to a failure of spontaneity and a striving for predictability—both of which miss the point, which is that anxiety creates the perfect environment for a horrific awareness of what could be, *god forbid*. Anxiety strips away the filters that make the unknown and uncontrollable a little bit more tolerable. It is thanks to these filters that we are able to get in our cars to drive to work, that we decide to have children, that we love one another. These filters protect us from being eaten up by the reality of our human condition, which is that chaos reigns, whether we think about it or not. It plays out in small, personal ways—like the fact that I can't know now how I will feel in three minutes, and what could change in that time (no matter the crystals, nor the lining up of shoes) fantastically or horrifically or in no meaningful way at all. And it plays out on the world stage—that, for instance, we are still coming to understand the effects of a global pandemic, the ram-ifications of which were unimaginable to most of us in early 2020. The anxiety we are protecting ourselves from is on the one hand en-tirely reasonable—it reflects the reality that life is finite—yet it is also a hindrance to vitality.

In *The Denial of Death*, anthropologist Ernest Becker writes about the ways in which we, as human beings, are impacted by the aware-ness of our own mortality, for better and for worse. Most of all, Becker writes about human anxiety in the face of death: "The idea of death, the fear of it, haunts the human animal like nothing else." In the 1980s, Becker's work inspired social psychologists Jeff Green-berg, Sheldon Solomon, and Tom Pyszczynski to develop terror management theory (TMT). TMT addresses the ways in which our awareness of our own eventual death relates to our views of the world, our behavior, and in particular, our self-esteem. According to TMT, anxiety is at the center of human experience, and self-esteem is an "anxiety buffer." With this buffer in place, we are able to go on with our lives without feeling constantly terrified by our awareness of our own mortality: "Self-esteem is the feeling that one is an object of pri-mary value in a meaningful universe. . . . From the perspective of terror management theory, people need self-esteem because it is the central mechanism for protecting individuals from the anxiety that awareness of their vulnerability and mortality would otherwise create." Faced, inevitably, by the limits of our own lives, we need something meaningful to hold on to.

Within the sphere of TMT research, there is powerful work be-ing done to support the intertwining of fears of death and obsessive-compulsive disorder. Research shows, for instance, that among people diagnosed with OCD, as fears of death increase, the severity of obsessive-compulsive disorder symptoms increases too. In the same vein, research has also found that mortality salience, which is to say, our conscious awareness of our own mortality, can impact our behavior. One study found that among people with OCD who engage in excessive washing behaviors (in this case, handwashing), when death is salient, washing increases. These participants literally used more soap to wash their hands. Though this link between OCD and fear of death is one that many people know in their bones, it can be difficult to point to, and to see this association play out in research is instructive. These findings allow us to work backward, and to understand more about ourselves and our anxieties.

Anxiety, obsessions, and compulsions teach us about our tenuous grasp on reason. But most of all, they teach us about the reasons hidden beneath the reasons. What is this fear, this worry, this dread, this urgency to act telling me? What is beneath the surface? I find that when you allow yourself to be curious, the answers aren't far off. Usually, the only thing that's really in the way is your belief in your own capacity to tolerate them. You will not drown in your fears. It will be a relief to speak them aloud or maybe even write them down, a relief felt not only in the mind but in the entirety of the body.

இ

In Greek mythology, Ananke is the goddess of compulsion and necessity, and the mother of the fates. She embodies that which we feel *must* be done, and that which feels inevitable. For decades, in psychiatric circles, Ananke's name was used in the term "anankastic personality disorder," which is now more commonly referred to as "obsessive-compulsive personality disorder" (OCPD) (the term "anankastia" remains in use in the *International Classification of Diseases*). Despite the similarity in their names, OCD and OCPD are distinct conditions with differing symptoms associated with them. Whereas individuals with OCPD tend to view their rigidly held beliefs as a reflection of how things *should*, in fact, be done, in OCD, rigidity is an undesired response to anxiety and fear. OCPD and OCD are sometimes differentiated in terms of their relationship to the self. OCPD is ego-syntonic, meaning that for the person experiencing it, it is in alignment with their sense of themselves. On the other hand, OCD is ego-dystonic, meaning that for the person experiencing it, it is out of sync with their sense of self, or put another way, they wish they could rid themselves of their symptoms. But despite these distinctions, OCPD and OCD share certain common threads. Both diagnoses ask us to think about the ways in which we feel under the sway of compulsion; of necessity; of how things should, need, to be; of feeling bound to our thoughts. Ananke reminds us about the place of flexibility in our thoughts and emotions—that these struggles are very, very old indeed. She is said to have been there when the universe was born.

Over the course of history, obsessions and compulsions have been subject to a range of frameworks of understanding. Because tendencies toward obsessionality and compulsivity are tightly linked to fears of wrongdoing, harm, and error, they have often manifested in the realms of religious belief and practice. In the seventeenth century, Robert Burton described people consumed with scrupulosity in his *Anatomy of Melancholy*, citing sixteenth-century physician Jason Pratensis: "They are troubled with scruples of conscience, distrusting God's mercies, think they shall go certainly to hell, the devil will have them, and make great lamentation." And though Burton's work is now four centuries old, in some respects, not much has changed. For many people experiencing anxiety, these ideas still hold today—in religious and secular contexts. Recent research emphasizes the different ways in which anxiety can be associated with religiosity, depending, above all, on the emotional nature of one's religious experience. Unsurprisingly, when religious beliefs are largely positive, including, for instance, faith and gratitude, people experience some protection from anxiety symptoms. On the other hand, when negative emotions are associated with one's religious beliefs, anxiety may actually increase.

Alongside this history of religious manifestations of anxiety comes the larger issue of whether the particular nature of the things we concern ourselves with, our idiosyncratic perseverations, matter for treatment. Whereas one person's anxiety might spike at the thought of a potential sin committed, another might perseverate about fears of accidental legal wrongdoing. Some clinicians and scholars argue that the content of obsessional, intrusive thoughts—for instance, "What if I accidentally run someone over with my car?" isn't important—that, essentially, the content of the thought could be anything, and even more so, that viewing intrusive thoughts as meaningful in and of themselves runs the risk of fueling them. If the thoughts themselves, rather than the manner of thinking, are given too much weight, the distress that they cause will only increase. But I've always struggled with the notion that the content doesn't matter. Where is it that our minds go?

Lawrence Price, MD, is a psychiatrist—both a clinician and a researcher—and an expert on OCD. I spoke with Price about his work and asked him whether or not he believes that the particular content of obsessive thoughts matters. He told me that it does, and also, it doesn't. On the one hand, at the level of the brain, when it comes to medication or neurological procedures to treat OCD, the content isn't so important. But in psychotherapy, surely the content does matter and needs to be addressed. Treatment for OCD emphasizes the importance of the ways that people interact with intrusive thoughts when they inevitably emerge. Let's return to "What if I accidentally run someone over with my car?" Rather than engaging with the thought actively by, for instance, trying to counteract it, argue with it, or dispute it ("But I've never had a car accident," "I always drive within the speed limit," "This thought is driving me crazy"), in treatment, patients learn to tolerate the thought and the accompanying discomfort without fighting it, and in this way, to let it pass. After the emotional intensity of these thoughts has dissipated, there is room for another kind of response. When you cultivate curiosity about the fear beneath the fear, you can reckon with the symbolic meaning of an obsessive thought rather than getting stuck in its literal content. Are we pulled toward fears of loss? Of destruction? Of contamination? Of death? In this way, the thoughts can become both less powerful and more meaningful.

Price is also one of the creators of the Yale-Brown Obsessive-Compulsive Scale, commonly known as the YBOCS, which has for years maintained its place as the leading tool for assessing OCD in clinical settings. The YBOCS includes questions like: "How much distress do your obsessive thoughts cause you?," "How would you feel if prevented from performing your compulsion(s)?," and "How much of an effort do you make to resist the compulsions?" The YBOCS is designed to be administered by a clinician through an extended interview. I've found that the YBOCS serves more than one function. Certainly, it evaluates the presence and extent of symptoms of OCD and contributes to diagnosis. But also, in administering the YBOCS, powerful conversations unfold. Patients think through aspects of their thoughts and behaviors that they may have previously avoided. The nature of the questions fosters curiosity and reflection about their experiences, rather than avoidance or shame.

I ask Price where he sees the future of treatment for OCD. We talk, first, about the ongoing importance of exposure and response prevention-based treatments (ERP). ERP, widely considered among the best treatments available for OCD, is used to treat a variety of forms of anxiety. Essentially, a patient is exposed to the situation (or thought or place) that makes them anxious and then does not engage in a response aimed at reducing that anxiety. The idea is that over time, they learn to tolerate the anxious feelings and thoughts associated with the situation, and little by little, the anxiety dissipates. A person with the intrusive thought, "What if I run someone over with my car by accident," who thus refuses to drive and will only use the bus or walk no matter the distance or weather or time of day, might begin by sitting in their car, turning on the ignition, and learning to tolerate the accompanying anxiety. The intrusive thought emerges— "What if I run someone over with my car by accident? My life would be destroyed. I would not be able to live with myself. My family's life would never be the same—nor would their family's life. I would go to prison." And so on. They might feel nauseated, begin to sweat, and feel the blood drain from their face. But rather than flee from the car, the thought, the anxiety itself, they would stay in their seat and allow the feelings to exist and then to pass. Uncomfortable at first, but survivable. Over time, they might then sit in the car, turn on the ignition, and drive down the block. Again, the thought, the anxiety. Uncomfortable at first, but survivable. Eventually, the goal would be to return to driving regularly without becoming overwhelmed.

ERP isn't perfect, but it is some of the best treatment we have to offer. On one hand, because it is usually targeted at specific anxieties, sometimes patients will work through one concern only to find that another, new one emerges. On the other hand, ERP, when used skillfully, with nuance, should drive at a tolerance of anxiety and uncertainty that extends beyond any one fear. Is it likely that you will run someone over with your car by accident? No. But is it possible? Of course. It can't be ruled out, and to move forward without anxiety taking over, we have to find a way to live with the reality that most of the time, we don't know for sure.

Price tells me, too, that he suspects the future of treatment for OCD will include psychedelics. Though research in this area is in its early days, studies suggest that psychedelics (like psilocybin) may indeed reduce symptoms of OCD and anxiety (as well as other conditions like depression, PTSD, and addiction). And while we have yet to fully untangle the neurological mechanisms at play, embedded in this work are principles of flexibility in our minds and bodies. In a recent paper on the role of psychedelics in mental health care, an international group of researchers argued that psychedelics are useful because they "destabilize fixed points or attractors, breaking reinforced patterns of thinking and behaving." A way toward flexibility.

I've said it before, and I'll say it again: we are only beginning to understand what it is that we are looking at. But what is clear is that whether it be through psychedelics or psychotherapy or through other means entirely, flexibility should, must, be on our minds.

⌾

Over the course of history, some of the words used to define "curiosity" have included:

> Carefulness, the application of care or attention . . .
>
> scrupulousness; exactness, accuracy . . .
>
> Care or attention carried to excess or unduly bestowed upon matters of inferior moment . . .
>
> subtlety . . .
>
> Desire to know or learn . . .
>
> —"Curiosity," *Oxford English Dictionary*

So curiosity can be "care or attention carried to excess," it can be "unduly bestowed"—but it can also be a "desire to know or learn." They are two sides of the same coin. When we are curious, we can come to know the places where we get stuck, and in this way, we can work toward flexibility.

When you call anxiety what it is, when you recognize its shape and its source, you can begin to counteract it. Daniel Siegel, a psychiatrist and expert on mindfulness, captures the benefits of articulating painful emotions with his phrase "name it to tame it." Research on affect labeling (putting words to feelings) and "emotional granularity" (doing so with specificity, a term introduced by neuroscientist Lisa Feldman Barrett) bears this out—studies show that articulating painful feelings is associated with a greater ability to regulate difficult emotions. We see emotional granularity play out in the ways we think and talk about our emotions—in the difference between describing feeling "stressed" and feeling, say, "overwhelmed, terrified of failure, and ill-equipped." Curiosity drives this kind of articulation, an inward curiosity about the specific nature of your own experience. In order to articulate emotions with depth, you ask questions of yourself, you dig deeper than you had before.

We all have particular constellations of feelings that we struggle with, and specificity guides us in organizing our internal experiences. When you put words to the nature of your distress, it becomes both more comprehensible and more approachable. When you name anxiety, perseveration slows, and you reassert your ability to think things through and to find your equilibrium. In this way, a space between yourself and your feeling is born, and little by little, it grows. It is not avoidance or denial—anyone who has tried to ignore anxiety knows it will only lead it to echo and expand. Instead, it is a roominess of thought that allows for reflection over hasty and potentially regrettable reactions. In this way, you cultivate a feeling of interest in your experience, one that extends beyond distress. This is the ultimate flexibility.

When I was writing my dissertation, I had a research mentor who, as a kind of praise, once told me that I take things very personally. I knew at the time that part of what he was conveying to me was that I take my responsibilities seriously, that they feel of personal import to me. And this is true. But also, he was telling me (as I'm sure he knew then) that perhaps I didn't need to feel things so personally. That it might be OK to relinquish some of that weight, to let go.

What he may not have known is that his words have stayed with me, and that years later, I continue to turn them over in my mind. They have helped me to find shape in a feeling that was once tied up in a nebulous kind of worry. That I take things so personally. That they feel so personal to me. That they are in some sense of my very person, a part of me. That I have, perhaps, a tender conscience. That this isn't solely pathological. That partly, I care. That there are worse things, but at the same time, taking things so personally can be a lot to hold on to. Through his gentle yet pointed language, I began to develop a sense of curiosity about this facet of my anxiety. I could be inquisitive, I could be full of care, about taking things personally, instead of just self-reproaching. And in this way, my curiosity began to shape a bit of space between myself and my anxiety. It became a way to drain the catastrophe away, and most of all, a way to think things through more flexibly. Now, I try to remind myself that when it comes to anxiety, curiosity is the opposite of rigidity. It is, in its very nature, counter to the sticky, perseverative thinking that takes us away from our loved ones and dims our days. It is through curiosity that our perspectives begin to shift, and sometimes we even change our minds, if even just for a moment.

Again and again, I'm drawn to the gray parts of life—the ambiguities, the unanswerable questions, and the uncertainty. Yet these are the very things that most pique my anxiety. We're drawn, above all, to the things that trouble us most, and whether we know it or not, it becomes our life's work to untangle them, to be curious about them. Our brains struggle with uncertainty, always wanting to place things into clean categories—like, in the case of anxiety, safe or dangerous, true or false. But when it comes to the brain, we are inevitably left to face how little we know. Blanket statements and attempts at oversimplification fail us. Findings do not always replicate. We are limited by our research methods and by our own minds. Ultimately, we have to learn to shift between these realities with flexibility and curiosity. To allow for the pragmatic and the linear, the discerning and skeptical, the curious and the awe-filled parts of ourselves to co-exist. This integration is what allows for truly powerful science, for reason with a backbone, and, too, for an acknowledgment of all that we have yet to learn, and may never know or understand. When it comes to understanding the brain and anxiety, our work has just begun. The body shows us, if we listen, that life goes on, until it doesn't. But along the way, when we feel stuck in ourselves and our uncertainties, curiosity, flexibility—they are a kind of resilience.

Part II

BLOOD

3.

BOUNDARIES AND
PERMEABILITY

Blood is a warning, its redness an alarm that
the casing of the body has been breached. That the
continuity of the tissue has been broken.

—Olga Tokarczuk, *Flights*

I n the brain, there is a wall of sorts, called the blood-brain barrier. This semipermeable collection of cells protects the brain from pathogens and other potentially detrimental intruders by allowing some substances entry while keeping others out. Our brains and blood are constantly interacting with each other, with the blood-brain barrier deciding what will be allowed in and what must stay away. In this way, it is a system of protection that is essential to human life—without it, the brain becomes vulnerable to all sorts of attacks, from infection to inflammation. This boundary is protected carefully and constantly, outside of our awareness. Its form and function even guide the creation of psychiatric medications (and other medications like anesthesia), which must be formulated to be capable of crossing the blood-brain barrier.

In our blood, another sort of boundary plays out, outside the realms of our control. How does my genetic inheritance shape my body? How does it impact the function of my organs and even my emotional life? What, for one reason or another, stays out and does not become a part of me? What of my blood comes from outside of myself—what traits, mutations, pathogens, what joys, what genetic future? And what develops within my own body, my own blood, as a product of my own experiences, the good and the bad? What then, might I pass on? These are difficult boundaries to locate.

The work of boundary keeping within our bodies and ourselves happens in the realms of our awareness too. We observe and construct boundaries in relationships of all kinds, and in the ways that we relate to our own experiences. Sometimes this is effortful—we work hard to establish limits in personal and professional contexts, or we hold them so strongly that we come to feel alone in the world. And when boundaries falter or fail, anxiety tends to emerge. In the midst of anxiety, whether a moment of doubt or a pervasive sense of dread, there are usually questions of boundaries to be asked and answered. What are we allowing in and what are we keeping out? How permeable are we to our environments and to the people around us? What sorts of lines do we draw in our own minds, and where do we place them? Our bodies show us this, across organ systems and in our emotional lives, again and again.

For much of human history, blood has held a steady position as a window into our insides, albeit in a variety of permutations. Blood has long been tied to life, death, and spirituality, as in Biblical times, and more recently, it has come to be understood in more practical terms as a substance whose role is to fuel the body in its entirety. In the classic *Gray's Anatomy*, first published in 1858, blood is described under the heading "The Nutritive Fluids" as "an opaque, rather viscid fluid, of a bright-red or scarlet color when it flows from the arteries, of a dark-red or purple color when it flows from the veins. It is salt to the taste, and has a peculiar faint odor." We see, across time and place, blood as a poetic force and a physical necessity, one with spiritual value, and with a strange smell too.

Blood was, for centuries, understood within the sphere of humoral theory. A cornerstone of medical history whose beginnings are now associated with Hippocrates's writings, humoral theory remained a part of medical practice into the nineteenth century. Humoral theory integrated the body and the world it exists within. In *The Greatest Benefit to Mankind: A Medical History of Humanity*, Roy Porter explains "'humoral medicine' stressed the analogies between the four elements of external nature (fire, water, air and earth) and the four humours or bodily fluids (blood, phlegm, choler or yellow bile and black bile), whose balance determined health." Blood had a special place in humoral theory—it was both one of the four humors and also a substance that contained the other three. According to this system of medicine, you will recall that balance in the body, and, too, the blood, was central to well-being, and imbalances between the four humors were the cause of all sorts of illness. Melancholy was thought to be the result of too much black bile in the body, and bloodletting, often via leeching, was a common treatment.

Today, we understand blood in different terms—we know that it is made up of plasma, which contains red blood cells, white blood cells, and platelets, each of which perform essential functions. Our red blood cells transport oxygen throughout our bodies, our white blood cells protect the body from illness, and platelets ensure proper clotting. The function and quantity of each of these elements is crucial to our health, indicative of wellness and potential disease. When we donate blood, we perform a lifesaving act of service. So much has changed, yet blood remains a place where boundaries blur, where dread and hope comingle.

Anxiety is in many ways written in our biological stars. Research consistently shows a strong genetic component to anxiety disorders. Anxiety runs in my family, so much so that we make a joke of it. There is comfort in the camaraderie, and relief in this tangible, phenotypic proof that anxiety courses through my veins. Relief because, to be honest, it is evidence that it can't simply be my fault. To be clear, I know better than to think this way, but here we are. Looking back over generations, I hear stories of grandparents and extended family members whose anxiety closely resembles my own. Avoiding risk, aiming for certainty, adhering to rules, finding comfort in order, fear of heights—these traits are as present as dark hair and brown eyes in my family tree. I wonder, when my son lines his rice cakes up in a row, if I've passed this curse on to him or if he will be spared. I ask myself if I can somehow protect him from this particular anguish, or if he will struggle in my way. It's too soon to say.

So we see that anxiety runs through bloodlines, yet it does so incompletely. The child of two anxious parents may go on to develop anxiety, but also, they may not. Conversely, the child of parents with minimal anxiety may struggle with a lifelong anxiety disorder. We know that the close family members of people with generalized anxiety disorder (and other common forms of anxiety) are some four to six times more likely to experience anxiety themselves than those without this family history. It is clear that genetics powerfully impact the transmission of anxiety disorders, yet they are far from straightforward.

In the world of genetics research, studies of twins were, for decades, the primary method for attempting to untangle questions of nature versus nurture that belie mental illness. Twin studies usually compare the outcomes of identical (monozygotic) twins to those of fraternal (dizygotic) twins. Identical twins have 100 percent (or in some instances nearly 100 percent) of their DNA in common, whereas dizygotic twins share about 50 percent of their DNA. Twins are, of course, the same age and usually raised in the same home environment. This means that researchers can look at the ways that genetics *in particular* may impact different health outcomes, rather than environmental forces that effect our mental health. Twin studies on anxiety disorders consistently find that a combination of genetic and environmental factors gives rise to anxiety disorders.

Now, cutting-edge technology is bringing us closer to anxiety's origins. Genome-wide association studies (GWAS), which look at vast amounts of genetic data, examine the human (or animal) genome to identify genetic variants associated with conditions or traits (like social anxiety or anxiety sensitivity). This work goes hand in hand with research that looks at the ways in which our well-being is shaped not by our genetics alone but rather by the interaction between our biology and our experiences. Diathesis-stress models of illness propose that disease comes about as a product of a combination of genetic and environmental factors. So, in the case of anxiety, you may have a genetic proclivity, due to a combination of genes, to particular anxious traits, and then be exposed to, say, high levels of stress in childhood, or a traumatic event, or a struggle with drug use, and subsequently develop an anxiety disorder. Or you may have a genetic proclivity to anxiety but, in the absence of these stressors, you may never develop an anxiety disorder of any kind. A recent, massive study looked at the ways that our genetics and our experiences interact and found, with a sample of thousands of participants, that exposure to stressful experiences (like loneliness and low levels of social support) can indeed increase genetic risk for anxiety as well as depression. When we think about the inheritance of anxiety disorders, all signs point to genetic risk rather than genetic guarantee.

Genetics research is also a powerful tool for understanding the relationships between different kinds of mental illness. Our diagnostic systems are based largely on assessing signs and symptoms—those aspects of mental illness that can be either observed by a clinician or reported by an individual, like, for instance, irritability, confusion, sadness, or worry. Thinking through the genetics of anxiety disorders, we come up against the limitations of the categorizations of anxiety that we depend on and which are so tightly woven throughout our systems of thinking about and treating these conditions. Recent research on the genetics of anxiety disorders is not only identifying genetic variations associated with the occurrence of anxiety but it is also beginning to link anxiety, post-traumatic stress disorder, depression, schizophrenia, and ADHD on a genetic basis.

One of the ways in which genetics research on anxiety and other kinds of mental illness strives to be of practical use is by guiding the development and selection of psychiatric medication for patients. The current (frustrating) reality of medication for anxiety disorders is that arriving at a good fit can involve a great deal of trial and error. Although sometimes the process is simple and the first medication a person tries dramatically improves their quality of life, it can also take time. A medication that works well for one person may not help another, and often there is no clear reason why. The weeks or even months of waiting for symptoms to improve can be agonizing.

In a burgeoning field known as pharmacogenomics, we are beginning to see the ways that genetics research may guide the treatment of anxiety disorders. Genetic testing is now being used to help psychiatrists and other prescribers to tailor medication choices with more specificity. This approach is known as genomically assisted prescribing. Psychiatrists can order genetic tests (this testing is done by taking a blood sample) for a specific patient and then use the results to select a medication that will, in theory, be a best fit for them. The goal here is for prescribers to be able to select medications that target the genetics of the patient in front of them, and in so doing, to treat patients more quickly and more effectively. In a study that compared using genomically assisted prescribing versus a typical medication selection process to treat depression and anxiety, more improvement in depression and anxiety was found for those who had been treated with a pharmacogenomics-based approach. But much remains to be seen—another recent study on the use of genomically assisted prescribing, in this case for children with diagnoses of anxiety, depression, or ADHD, found that genomically assisted prescribing seemed to improve treatment outcomes for children with ADHD but not for children with anxiety or depression.

Will pharmacogenomics become a household term, a standard practice in the coming years? These tests may very well become just as commonplace as all sorts of genetic testing we now participate in, like the testing we use to learn about our ancestry or even the ancestry of our pets. But although pharmacogenomics are a step toward more effective decision-making, they are an imperfect offering at best. Current research demonstrates that there are a number of factors at play in limiting the use of pharmacogenomics—among them, limited high-quality research on their utility and limited training for providers in how to actually utilize these tools.

When things become common, it's easy to forget their significance. But genetic testing is a profound view inside ourselves, one whose ramifications are only just beginning to show themselves. Anxiety forces us to face the boundaries between what we can and cannot know, what we can and cannot be sure of—and genetic testing pushes up against these lines. Before genetic testing became routine, or at least somewhat more accessible, it was as though there were a solid line within the body, a helpful line, one that divided what could be known from what we just don't get to know. You could know your cholesterol levels or your blood pressure or your blood sugar, but you could not know your odds of inheriting a terminal illness from your parent or of passing that illness on to your child. And as much as genetic testing can be, and often is, an incredibly powerful, lifesaving tool for early detection and disease prevention, in some ways, the old line felt good, or at least easier. I recall a patient who began therapy after her mother was diagnosed with a life-altering genetic illness. The patient had recently given birth and was terrified that she might develop the same condition as her mother or, worse, have passed it down to her child. On one hand, she felt a sense of urgency to be tested as soon as possible, in the hopes that she would receive comforting news. On the other hand, though, she was terrified to undergo the testing, terrified of what it might portend. The invitation, indeed the choice to know more—this is where anxiety grows.

When we are faced with the opportunity to see more deeply inside our bodies, we come up against questions not only of what we want to know about ourselves but also of what we resist knowing. And, it turns out, the answer is often: quite a lot. This happens in psychotherapy, too, a process that, broadly speaking, aims to increase self-knowledge and thus improve one's quality of life. You might begin to engage, for the first time, in a conversation about a painful pattern in your romantic relationships that you can't seem to extricate yourself from, but find yourself shutting it down. Or you might turn away from an observation about your behavior that feels, at its core, true, yet too overwhelming to examine. In their own ways, therapy and genetic testing can evoke a fear of what one might learn and a powerful impulse to look away. Sometimes, the idea of knowing the contents of one's insides is more appealing in the abstract than it is in reality. Seeing yourself can be painful.

The thought of sending a vial of my saliva off in the mail for a broad swath of genetic testing makes me feel a bit sick. As much as I'm intrigued by the idea of confirming (or, more intriguingly, being surprised by) my heritage, I know that the horror I would experience were I to learn about diseases that could be waiting for me in the future, without any clear course for prevention, would, for me, override any gains. I already have a clear idea of the illnesses that run in my family, and I am acutely aware of their associated risks. To subject myself to this kind of vast genetic testing would almost certainly be an invitation for decades of worry about a future that I can neither change nor fully predict. Genetics aren't always fate.

When I was pregnant, I underwent the standard New York City battery of genetic tests—which is to say, probably far more extensive than the testing that is typical elsewhere in the United States. Through this process, I learned that I was a genetic carrier for a couple of improbable conditions, and that our son would be safe from them as long as my husband wasn't a carrier too. This information was presented to me in a matter-of-fact, unconcerned manner—yet it initially had me spinning. And as much as I was reassured to learn that these conditions were not only unlikely but also not life threatening, and that a happy life could be lived with them, I felt myself being stretched. It was as though my anxiety, and more specifically my ability to tolerate uncertainty with some degree of calm, was undergoing a new sort of challenge. I wanted the genetics counselor to be able to give me (impossibly) clear answers, but I also knew that even if they did, it wouldn't provide me with what I was really after—which was a guarantee that my child would be healthy and happy, and that he would not suffer. There is, of course, no such thing.

I remember two conversations with my parents during this period, in which I expressed my fears for my baby, and they both, independently of each other, pointed out to me that this wrestling with uncertainty, this particular kind of anxiety, this was an unavoidable part of parenthood, and that it would be a fixture in my life from here on out. It was also during this time that I came to understand that this would be my first of many struggles with the question of what we, what I, pass along to our offspring—not just through our blood but also through our own histories and our ways of relating to the world.

We see different kinds of inheritance and transmission at play in our families—those traits that seem to be transmitted through bloodlines, and also the ways that our patterns of behavior are impacted by the experiences of those who came before us and can impact the generations that follow us. It happens in memorable moments—in times of decision, joy, and tragedy—and also in the minutia of everyday life. This isn't something we can (yet) pinpoint directly in the blood, yet more and more evidence is demonstrating that it is not just DNA but experience, too, that exists in the body, passed along like so many other traits.

During one of our many split-second disputes about whether or not to cross the street at a yellow light, I explained to my husband that there needed to be enough time to account for the possibility that I could trip and fall while in the crosswalk. In the moment, this seemed to me like a reasonable precaution—like planning ahead, getting in front of a problem. Yet he found it absurd that this would be something I would consider. And as I heard myself, my logic sounded, indeed, absurd. In moments of contrast, we tend to come up against our own anxiety. We see the gap between our response and that of another person. This happens in childhood and adolescence as we witness and push up against our family's limits and those of other households, and it continues into adulthood, at work, in relationships. Seeing my logic, myself, through my husband's eyes, I am reminded of how anxiety can infiltrate small moments, and, if unchecked, it can insidiously shape our days. Just as life experiences, whether in childhood or later on, can teach or otherwise give rise to anxiety, experience can also jostle anxiety out of its usual place, and can be a chance to see it anew.

We are just beginning to understand the conditions under which our genetics and our experiences impact the form and degree of our anxieties. When we know our struggles deeply, we can begin to step outside cycles of repetition with more flexibility. And we can think more effectively about prevention. If a proclivity exists in one's family, what skills, what attitudes might we cultivate? When I hear myself saying DON'T to my son—DON'T swing too high, DON'T touch that leaf, DON'T . . . I think about how he will, in years to come, make sense of his own upbringing. Will he think his mother worried too much? Probably. And while it's nice to imagine that becoming aware of one's own anxiety will make it possible to entirely avoid the anxious behaviors that a child might observe and repeat, this is far more easily said than done. Even with introspection, with therapy, with treatment, we can't escape ourselves. Our own struggles, which we didn't lick off the street, inevitably filter down, in one way or another, to our children. But mostly, people are doing their best, and doing so with immense love. This filters down too.

〰

The interactions that take place between anxiety and blood extend far beyond genetics. Though there is no doubt in my mind that the idiosyncratic collections of traits that we do and do not inherit through genetic means have powerful implications for our experience of anxiety, this is the tip of the iceberg. Every day, our blood, a dynamic system, interacts with circumstance. These circumstances form a kind of conversation between anxiety and the blood.

That our blood changes in response to fear and anxiety is a very old phenomenon—and it has contributed hugely to our survival. Our blood vessels constrict in "fight-or-flight" states, and blood pressure increases. This is all for good reason—the body's logic is that by getting blood to our extremities, we are ready to fight or to run. And blood clots more efficiently when we are afraid. As the body prepares for a fight, it also prepares for blood loss. Indeed, another instance in which the blood clots more readily is during pregnancy— and this, too, is because the body is preparing for the loss of blood that comes with giving birth. So the body holds on to its blood with an especially tight grip when it anticipates attack or injury. But the body is imperfectly calibrated, and hypercoagulation (increased clotting of the blood) is of little use in the face of most modern stressors. It does you no good when work is stressful, or when you experience family conflict or are stuck in traffic. Sometimes, changes in the blood in response to stress can become harmful, contributing to unnecessary clotting of the blood. The body's efforts to protect us from blood loss may also, in some circumstances, contribute to the development of heart disease—particularly for people with preexisting heart conditions. Acute stress can lead to hypercoagulability, and for some people this may lead to lasting damage to the circulatory system and contribute to dangerous conditions like heart attacks.

Our bodies work hard to protect us. But there is always a cost.

Across medical disciplines, research is accumulating that points toward the importance of inflammation in understanding a wide range of disease processes. Bear in mind, inflammation is intended to protect the body from harm. It is the result of our immune system responding to an actual or perceived threat. If, for instance, you trip and fall onto your knee, the swelling in the area is inflammation doing its work. The blood vessels dilate, and extra oxygen is sent to the wound. Specialized white blood cells (which are part of the immune system) go to the area of the wound to help to reduce the risk of infection. So inflammation has its necessary place, yet in excess, inflammation becomes a problem. In this way, it is not so different from anxiety. These bodily strains, like the impaired functioning of the blood, have cumulative effects that we are only at the start of understanding.

While inflammation can occur in any number of places in the body, one of our best ways to assess whether it is happening and to what degree is through inflammatory markers that are measured in the blood. When I first began to learn about inflammation and its wide-ranging impact on well-being years ago, it struck me as suspect. Inflammation seemed to become an overarching explanation for an endless list of health problems, and it sounded more like a marketing strategy for dietary supplements and anti-inflammatory cookbooks that looked like they'd been pumped out of a factory than much of an explanation for what ails us. But I've come to believe that when it comes to understanding anxiety (and so many other mental health conditions), inflammation merits the attention that it is getting.

Some research shows that there can be increases in inflammatory markers in the body during times of anxiety and depression—though it's important to bear in mind that data is only beginning to accumulate in this area and it isn't conclusive. One meta-analysis found increased pro-inflammatory cytokines in people with PTSD, but not in those with OCD or an anxiety disorder. Another meta-analysis on the link between generalized anxiety disorder and inflammation pointed toward a relationship between the two but also noted that it remains to be seen whether or not inflammation is a *cause* of generalized anxiety disorder. Remarkably, there is a growing body of research showing that the class of antidepressants called selective serotonin reuptake inhibitors (SSRIs), a group of psychiatric medications that includes well-known medications like Prozac, Zoloft, and Lexapro, that, as you recall, are commonly used to treat anxiety and depression, may actually have anti-inflammatory effects. If research in this area continues to bear out, it may be that when SSRIs reduce symptoms of anxiety and depression, they do so, at least in part, by reducing inflammation in the body. Though these findings are, remember, imperfect, not set in stone, they are staggering. Reading clinical research can feel like looking into the future—because it inevitably takes time for scientific findings to make their way into practice, and then into the mainstream. If, eventually, the scientific and clinical communities come to a consensus that inflammation is a central factor in the development and subsequent treatment of anxiety, this could mark a sea change in psychology and psychiatry. It could, of course, shift how we think about the role of SSRIs in modern medicine, but even more so, it could change the way we think about the roots of anxiety itself.

Some studies have also begun to explore the ways that techniques we use to manage difficult emotions may impact the inflammatory system and our health more broadly. Psychologist Megan Renna has proposed a model (the biobehavioral model of negative emotionality) that describes the connection between so-called negative emotions (like anxiety) and inflammation. Renna emphasizes that although negative emotions can give rise to bodily responses like inflammation, which can, as we know, be harmful for our health, we do have some recourse. Renna argues that emotion regulation is the pivotal point in this process—which is to say, if we learn to respond to difficult times adaptively, we can mitigate the risk of bodily harm through mechanisms like inflammation, whereas if we respond in harmful ways, we may increase the odds of ongoing damage to the body. We see, again and again, the ways in which our emotional experiences and our bodies are, undeniably, in constant interaction.

In psychological and psychiatric research, scar models look at the ways that an experience of mental illness, like generalized anxiety disorder or a major depressive episode, can bring about lasting changes in the body, leaving a kind of scar behind. A burgeoning scar model and accompanying evidence propose that experiences of anxiety and depression may be linked to future problems with executive functioning, which includes crucial brain functions like planning, short-term memory, and attention. And it turns out that inflammation is at play in the link between anxiety and depression and problems with executive functioning. In a recent study, researchers first looked at psychiatric symptoms, like anxiety and depression, among adults in the United States. Then, they looked at measurements of inflammation levels taken two months later, followed by measures of executive functioning taken eighteen months after that.

Higher levels of anxiety and depression were related to an upswing in inflammation, and that upswing in inflammation was related to problems with executive functioning at the final stage in the study. The same research team conducted another study in which they looked at data captured over an eighteen-year period. Again, they found that depression and anxiety were linked to subsequent inflammation, which was then found to be related to later declines in executive functioning.

The implications of this research are staggering. By pinpointing a chain of events that can begin with anxiety, followed by inflammation, and then future cognitive decline, there is great preventative potential. I spoke to Nur Hani Zainal, PhD, a postdoctoral research associate at Harvard Medical School and coauthor of these studies, about this work and especially about the ways in which scar models may help us to intervene in order to reduce the negative effects of anxiety and inflammation on the body over time. Zainal emphasized the importance of sleep and physical activity in protecting the brain, and pointed out that physical activity can be loosely defined, including lower-impact exercise like walking. Zainal also pointed to the value of combining psychotherapy, medication, and behavioral changes (like physical activity) when anxiety is severe, to mitigate risks of long-term cognitive effects following anxiety and inflammation. We also spoke about the future of scar theory and anxiety. What might be possible if we, as a society, were to take seriously this idea that there are real consequences to a lack of treatment for conditions like anxiety, consequences that can have major impact on well-being over time? Perhaps we would devote greater resources to mental health from the get-go, instead of waiting for things to unravel. As we spoke, I thought, too, about the ways in which the boundaries that we imagine between the working of our bodies and our minds are false. We cannot truly separate anxiety from inflammation, or physical activity from mental health—they move together. We can't treat the mind properly when we leave the body behind.

℘

I try to notice plasticity wherever I can. When, for instance, my son hesitates to climb a ladder on the playground, I think of the fear of heights that runs in my family—a fear that is heritable. I watch, I notice, and sometimes I try to quell this anxiety before it grows stronger. After all, my blood is coursing through his veins. But on the other hand, my experience isn't his experience. We don't want to see ourselves in our children so much that we miss them. So much is possible, so much can change.

In these moments, I think of blood and inheritance and boundaries—about the lines between ourselves and those we love and who love us. If I fail to see the space between myself and my son, between me and the generation that follows me, or between me and the generation that came before, I'm inadvertently inhibiting growth and progress—I'm missing the boundary. And when we talk about anxiety, we are inevitably talking about boundaries. About the lines, however blurry, between oneself and others, between too much and not enough, and about the ways in which we are permeable to the world. When our boundaries are too weak, we become permeable to fears and experiences that are not our own. We lose track of the anxieties that belong to ourselves and those that belong elsewhere, and in doing so, we lose our capacity to see things as they are. And lest it sound like boundaries discourage empathy, it is quite the opposite. With good boundaries, we can see ourselves and others more clearly, and in this way, we become more capable of authentic empathy.

Here are some of the illnesses in which the blood-brain barrier, that ultimate boundary, can falter: Alzheimer's disease. Dementia. Strokes. And even in the absence of these devastations, inevitably, as we age, the blood-brain barrier loses some of its effectiveness. We see the physical and emotional consequences of our body's boundaries weakening. But no matter our age, our boundaries are, inevitably, imperfect, at times permeable, as they should be. Yet they are protections that we must come to know. And when our blood clots, it, too, forms a protective boundary between our bodies and the world. It forms a scab, a reminder, at least for a while, of the ways that boundaries shift and change in the body—of how sometimes we are too permeable, but also, we heal.

4.

A FORCE TO BE
RECKONED WITH

His body and his limbs were brazen and
invulnerable, except at one point: under a sinew by
his ankle there was a blood-red vein protected only
by a thin skin which to him meant life or death.

—Apollonius of Rhodes, *The Voyage of Argo*

B lood contains tension. It belongs to our insides, but it is also a
visible part of ordinary life. A paper cut, teeth flossed too
harshly, the birth of a child—blood is created and flows constantly in the body, and when it emerges, it is bright and urgent.
Children respond with horror at the sight of a tiny wound, a loss of
blood with no medical consequences to speak of. A part of the body
that can so easily escape its confines must be very powerful indeed.

Blood, as an agent of health and illness, evokes anxiety because it
reminds us that much is happening, unseen and well outside the
realms of our control, inside our bodies. Just as people have always

understood the dangers of losing blood, so, too, have its curative properties long been a part of medicine. History shows us that we have always been attempting to harness our blood, and in doing so, to understand and maybe even control our beginnings and our endings. Attempts at blood transfusions date back at least to the seventeenth century. We see, too, instances of people attempting to consume and literally incorporate blood as a form of treatment for a range of ailments. In his fascinating book on vampires, Nick Groom details instances of blood consumption and blood use as medical treatment: "Pliny recorded epileptics drinking the warm blood of dying gladiators; the medieval mystic Hildegard of Bingen recommended baths of menstrual blood (*sanguis menstruus*) to cure leprosy—a belief that lasted for centuries. . . . The English College of Physicians included 'mummy, human blood, and human skull' in their official pharmacopoeia of 1618." Blood has always operated at the crossroads of illness and treatment—as both problem and solution. Too much of it was thought to cause illness, yet in some contexts it was believed to be curative. So, too, bloodlike substances have been highly valued for their medicinal uses for much of human history. The dragon blood tree, *Dracaena cinnabari,* is found on the Yemeni island of Socotra, and it (along with some of its cousins) is known for its bloodlike red sap and its curative properties. Dragon's blood has been used to treat conditions as far ranging as fever, ulcers, and loose teeth, and it has been used to encourage wound healing and stop hemorrhaging. These days, you can find it easily, in its liquid form, among the crystals and tarot cards in so-called metaphysical shops. And in laboratory settings, research over recent decades has made clear the chemical properties of dragon sap that underlie its medical utility, something that people around the world have understood for centuries. So we see that blood and its likenesses have long been understood as a reminder of the inevitability of death, but also, as a font of vitality.

In the seventeenth century, William Harvey, an English physician who had trained in Italy, discovered the mechanisms by which blood circulates throughout the body. Harvey wrote about his findings in no uncertain terms: "It is absolutely necessary to conclude that the blood in the animal body is impelled in a circle and is in a state of ceaseless motion." The principle of circulation of the blood throughout the body marked a monumental shift in Western medicine. This was a force of life that was, thanks to the heart, moving perpetually about the body. Even now, research is highlighting the importance of blood circulation to the brain in particular for neurological health—for example, to reduce the risk of dementia.

Medicinal practices around the world have, for thousands of years, reflected the importance of moving other kinds of life forces around the body. We see these principles in, for instance, Chinese medicine and Japanese medicine, in acupuncture and Reiki, respectively. Sanskrit texts refer to prana, a multidimensional life force that moves through the world and the body too. These practices have in common an interest in working against stagnation and toward a circulation of energy, of life itself, as a means of promoting health and healing in the physical and emotional realms. In my own daily life, when I go for a run, I imagine my blood circulating throughout my brain, steadfast and nutritive, a force of life.

Anxiety feels, more often than not, like a problem that requires solving, a kind of suffering that we wish to eliminate rather than examine. But in the right light, anxiety can lead us toward the answers to some of the questions we hold most closely. Our anxieties can become a powerful source of information—about the worries and fears that plague us, yes, and also about the things we desire that have yet to unfold. In this way, anxiety is malleable—it can manifest as dread that overwhelms the body, but it can also become a vital, generative force.

When I was a child, prone to rumination about health problems, my mother would remind me that "common things are common." Growing pains were common—cancer of the leg in small children was not. She had learned this phrase from her father, who was a physician, so it had a certain weight given my fears. I remember holding on to this idea, repeating it in my mind: Of course! Common things are common! This is reasonable. With this hit of logic, a sense of calm would wash over my body, if briefly. My heart rate would slow, my stomach would settle. Indeed, it was most likely that my fears were unfounded, or at the very least, overblown. But inevitably, before much time had passed, the doubt would creep back in. After all, common things are indeed common, but uncommon things are possible too.

We always want to know where we stand. I am healthy, or this is who I am, where I am from. But most often, the information available to us is imperfect, incomplete at best. At the crossroads of anxiety and the body is health anxiety. Health and, conversely, illness, are a perfect petri dish for anxiety to expand in—because our bodies are never entirely knowable. We are in a state of constant change, and with rare exceptions, we don't get to see our insides (nor would most of us know what to make of them even if we could). We look to blood to provide essential information about the state of our health, and in a sense, about the state of our future. But normal bloodwork at an annual physical does not eliminate the possibility of being diagnosed with a fatal illness six months later. This is, of course, the reality of being alive—our bodies do not work perfectly—yet for some, this is a painful uncertainty to accept. In this way, anxiety regarding the state of one's body gets right at anxiety's intractable core: nothing is certain, except that all of us will one day die. This bears out in data—health anxiety is consistently associated with difficulty tolerating uncertainty. In a google rabbit hole (which, in a Freudian moment, I mistyped as "rabbithold," certainly more what it feels like), I happen upon numan.com, a company offering what they call the "Fear Nothing Blood Test."

In cases of health anxiety, a great deal of energy is subsumed by concerns about symptoms and diagnoses. Time is spent checking the body for problematic changes, attending unnecessary appointments, and attention is diverted away from other parts of life. Instead of a baseline sense of bodily trust, there is bodily dread. The literal state of the body becomes an object of hyperfocus, when, in fact, there are usually larger questions at hand—questions like: *Will everything I care about, including my body, be taken from me? How would I cope? But what about my child?*

Health anxiety is nothing new—in fact, it is a very old condition, and one that is probably best documented in Burton's *The Anatomy of Melancholy*. He wrote, "Yet their bodies are out of tune, they suspect some part or other to be amiss, now their head aches, heart, stomach, spleen . . . they shall surely have this or that disease." The current (much drier) diagnosis of illness anxiety disorder, according to DSM-5 criteria includes: "preoccupation with having or acquiring a serious illness" and "a high level of anxiety about health, and the individual is easily alarmed about personal health status." Reading these two descriptions of what we now call health anxiety alongside each other, though they are separated by four centuries, we see that our bodies have always been, will always be, a place where anxiety dwells. Burton's references to headaches and problems with the stomach would be equally apt today, and the DSM-5's point that people with health anxiety are "easily alarmed about personal health status," though not so inspired, could just as well describe the people Burton referred to. We are stuck with ourselves, with our bodies, in all their imperfection and mortality, and there is no kind of human progress that will take that away. Anxiety associated with our bodily well-being raises questions for us all: Where do our energy and our attention (those most vital life-forces) go when we are anxious? And then, when they feel stuck in our bodies unnecessarily, where else might they be directed? What, really, is safety, and what is danger? How do we take care of ourselves while also accepting the uncertainty that is inherent in being alive? These are questions that underlie all sorts of anxiety, beginning with those survival instincts that are essential to our physiology.

When anxiety is high and the space between panic and calm feels narrow, it can be difficult to separate the problems and worries that need to be acted upon swiftly and those that need, instead, to be tolerated, lived with, and reevaluated in the future. It goes something like this: Should I get that bump on my arm looked at *right now*; is this urgent? Or, should I instead wait a few days to see if it goes away on its own? Will my day be derailed by this thought, or can I set it aside and attend to it in due course? What, in this instance, is due course? In the time it takes to notice some aberration, whether tiny or significant, health anxiety can take over one's mood, and suddenly energy is redirected to what feels like a crisis. This is because health anxiety creates a sense of being in danger, and an urge to find safety immediately. Alternatively: A friend of mine recently mentioned, in passing, a new asymmetry that she had noticed in one of her legs—one that neither she nor I knew anything about or could explain away as just fine or something to be concerned about. She looked me in the eyes and said, with total sincerity, "I'm really scared." And then, seamlessly, she went on to say how excited she was about her new apartment. I don't think she was avoiding the issue—rather, I think she was able to simultaneously hold this self-professed fear, this uncertainty about the workings of her body, alongside a sense of promise for the future. She could be alarmed without being consumed. The tone of her experience was not overshadowed by dread of the unknown.

We know that we are built to seek safety, and surely there are worse things. But perceptions of safety vary dramatically, and anxiety is associated with perceptions of danger where danger is not. The term "safety behavior" refers to things we do in the context of anxiety to prevent feared outcomes—for instance, checking repeatedly that a door is locked, or being sure to always sit near an exit in public spaces. But safety behaviors can be difficult to parse because sometimes they can seem reasonable, even advisable, out of context. Frequency and emotionality become the dividing lines between what is a safety behavior and what isn't. Is the behavior excessive? And, most of all, what is the emotionality attached to the behavior? If you schedule an annual mammogram, this is healthy and important. But if you schedule three unwarranted breast exams a year, just in case, this is a safety behavior. And what about the emotionality attached to it, the worry? What about the mental preparation for catastrophe? Research shows that although safety behaviors are a means to reduce anxiety, they tend to work alongside anxiety rather than providing any real, lasting relief.

So where is the line between safety behaviors and reasonable caution? I can say, advise, believe that it has to do with frequency and emotionality. But truthfully, it remains foggy. This is the pull of health anxiety—it resists clear delineation. What is truly necessary? Is a doctor's appointment unnecessary because it turns out that you aren't dying? That would be an absurd line to draw. In 1994, in a now classic paper titled "Generalized Anxiety Disorder (GAD) as an Unsuccessful Search for Safety," Sheila Woody and Stanley Rachman describe the process and aims of psychotherapy for anxiety, explaining that "the means of achieving safety are internalized and always available. In essence, the safety network is expanded to include the self." This is a beautiful description of treatment gone right, and it captures precisely the sort of distress that safety behaviors are an attempt to alleviate. When you are anxious, your sense of safety doesn't feel dependable, it doesn't feel entirely yours to call upon. Even your own body feels like a threat. It's no surprise, then, that in this way, health anxiety becomes a vortex into which energy is drawn.

In recent history, we've begun to see a new manifestation of health anxiety taking place, like so much of modern life, on the internet. The term "cyberchondria" refers to illness anxiety that is accompanied with repeatedly, compulsively even, seeking out information about one's health on the internet, which tends to contribute to further anxiety and is associated with reassurance seeking, difficulty tolerating uncertainty, and compulsivity. In clinical conversations, we sometimes refer to this as another kind of "GAD"—rather than generalized anxiety disorder, "google-induced anxiety disorder." A recent meta-analysis argues that cyberchondria is a type of safety behavior. These findings align with my clinical experience—the urge to google a health concern is, at its core, a wish for reassurance, a wish to be told that death is not imminent, that you are fundamentally OK, that you are safe and sound. You've simply taken on a new source—rather than a doctor or a friend, the internet. But the internet is terrible at providing reassurance—because it is fickle, untrustworthy, and worst of all, bottomless. And as much as we may know better, the internet is always right there, at our fingertips, no appointment required. And it does not chastise us or leave us embarrassed by our bodies or our doubts. Worst of all, when we search for information about our health and our bodies online, we tend to do it alone. There is no human response, no conversation, just a silent scream.

Thinking about health anxiety and the layers of fear that it contains, I wonder about comfort and where to find it, or better yet, how to create it. And I wonder about how to preserve that energy within us all, to keep it for the places where it belongs, the enriching places. I find a certain relief in hearing good medical providers talk about death. Certainly, they are trained to understand disease and its effects on the body, but more than that, it is their tone. They look at death head-on, with a good dose of wisdom and a bigger dose of warmth. Maybe, after years of being privy to cure and death both, they accept that the body can only be known and controlled to a point, because our bodies function to varying degrees, until they don't. Usually, each passing day isn't the end of the world. Usually, all is not lost. And alongside this capacity, I find that there is something else, something more difficult to pin down: they face these realities every day, but also, they do other things. They take care of their kids. They watch the game. They read books. Their acceptance creates space for life—for quotidian pleasure and curiosity and joy—and in this way, their energy is malleable.

I am not suggesting that we ignore concerns about our health. It bears mentioning that the matter of how to think through the attention we direct toward the state of our bodies exists within the larger context of a long-standing (and, it seems, perpetually ongoing) history of inequity in our health-care system, in which the health and the pain of all people are not treated equally. The health concerns of people of color and women are too often ignored, underresearched, and misattributed to anxiety. Pain is minimized and considered unreasonable or chalked up to needless complaining. These are profoundly harmful and well-documented aspects of the history and present day of medicine, and ones that we cannot ignore when we think about the dynamics at play when people experience health anxiety.

There is a risk of grave harm when people's experiences of changes and pain in their bodies are wrongly ignored. Heart disease, whose symptoms are easily minimized as anxiety, remains underdiagnosed and causes more deaths among women in the United States than any other condition. In *Unwell Women,* Elinor Cleghorn writes, "Women are more likely to be offered minor tranquilizers and antidepressants than analgesic pain medication. . . . And women's pain is much more likely to be seen as having an emotional or psychological cause, rather than a bodily or biological one." We should not stop noticing changes in our bodies, nor should we stop asking questions.

In a paper on the impact of structural racism on well-being, social epidemiologist Zinzi D. Bailey and colleagues explain that "structural racism has had a substantial role in shaping the distribution of social determinants of health and the population health profile of the USA, including persistent health inequities," and they describe the particular negative effects of structural racism on health, from symptoms of mental illness to trouble sleeping to inflammation. Experiences with health-care providers, and the provision of care by health-care providers, should always be seen in the context of the reality of inequity that we live in.

When it comes to anxiety about one's health, in circumstances in which anxiety is in fact the primary matter at hand, relief can come in the form of learning to experience questions and uncertainties differently. Although people with illness anxiety disorder will likely always wrestle with a higher degree of concern around bodily changes than others, over time and with practice, it is possible to pay attention to them in a new way: thoughtfully, but without panic, without being consumed by some anticipated disaster. In this spirit, and bearing in mind existing research on the role of attention in anxiety, there is a growing body of work on the relationship between health anxiety in particular and attention. We know that anxiety is associated with heightened attention to threat—and a recent meta-analysis found evidence that people with health anxiety devote increased attention to information that contains threats to health specifically. They also found that people with health anxiety *maintain* attention for health threats more so than those without health anxiety. So we see that health anxiety is associated with a movement of attention toward certain kinds of threat, and also that attention seems to get stuck there. Another recent study found that some people with health anxiety controlled their attention in order to *avoid* uncertainty-related content. We know that avoidance tends to perpetuate anxiety of all kinds. And although this may sound, at first glance, like research that emphasizes the value of developing control over one's attention, this can backfire when control results in avoidance. So it seems that health anxiety and attention can move together, and in this way, a great deal of cognitive resources—of energy, of that force within that could be put to good use—are misdirected and consumed, drawn away from more generative places.

⳥

These days, when we think of blood, we tend to think of injury and death—of what happens at the end. But blood is also essential to our beginnings. In the midst of giving birth to my son, a doctor shouted to the medical students surrounding her, "She's a bleeder!" I couldn't see the blood myself, and I didn't pay much attention to the remark at the time. I remember someone cleaning up the room as I recovered, and I wondered if birth was always so bloody. In keeping with some of my unusual childhood interests, in middle school I had been fascinated by *A Baby Story* on TLC and watched it weekly. This early reality show was all about pregnancy and birth, and it included what had seemed to me at the time to be graphic footage of child-birth, none of which had included so much blood. I suppose I filed the word "bleeder" away in my mind, but later, after things were calm and quiet, my husband told me how terrifying all the blood had been. He said that there was so much of it that it hardly seemed real, that my blood had been splashed all over the doctors' gowns and all over the delivery room. I was struck by his reaction—it was so unlike him—but I also wondered if he was making a big deal out of nothing. There was our son, full of life, so much beginning, but then, so much blood—and soon, there it was, too: a hint of fear, of the endings that in another time in history, in another place in the world, might have befallen us that day.

A year or so later, I started to notice bruising on my legs, though I couldn't remember having bumped into anything. The first few times these bruises appeared, I tried to ignore them. I told myself that I must have simply forgotten what happened in the midst of my busy days. After all, with a toddler learning to walk, and me often playing with him on our wooden living-room floor, maybe I shouldn't have been at all surprised to be a little bit banged up. Plus, I told my-self, I'm clumsy and always have been, so why was I alarmed by a few bruises? Maybe this was to be expected. Maybe this was more than enough information. I moved between wanting a clear expla-nation for what I was seeing and trying to reason myself out of my worst fears. Time passed, but still it didn't settle within me. Little by little, my childhood fear of fatal illnesses—of leukemia—began to creep out of decades of dormancy and back into my mind.

Were my concerns excessive? Was I catastrophizing, or was I rightly paying attention to my body by trusting myself to notice a change and following my instincts? A familiar thought returned: If I were to miss, or worse yet, to ignore something that turned out to be medically important, something with real ramifications, I would not be able to forgive myself. Only this time around, it was different—my son and his well-being were now at the front of my mind. Was my concern about my bodily health and my desire for an explanation a safety behavior to be understood and worked through? Or simply a safe behavior? Or both?

I decided to go to the doctor. I was tired of the internal back-and-forth. It felt like a waste of my time and my energy, especially in a situation in which answers might actually exist. As I sat in the doctor's waiting room, I noticed myself trying to be calm, and then, in her office, I heard myself downplaying my concerns. I said that I was often playing with my son on the wooden floor of our apartment, that maybe that was all there was to it. Of course, once I was there, none of what I said had much bearing on what would need to be done. The doctor ordered some blood work, and days later, I learned that my blood just clots a bit more slowly than is typical. And that there was no indication of leukemia.

Soon after, my doctor called me (which I found alarming in and of itself) and recommended that we repeat the blood work, just in case. It will come as no surprise that I wanted to know precisely what cases we were looking out for and how urgent this was. I had just moved far from home and had barely gotten my bearings. Could the blood work wait a few months? So it came as a great relief when she told me that this wasn't urgent, and that it could certainly wait. I reminded myself that urgent and important are not the same thing.

Around this time, COVID changed everything. For months, I,

like so many of us, barely left my home and avoided unnecessary medical appointments. Months went by, maybe a year. I wondered about the bruises sometimes, and my desire for answers. The matter of getting the blood work repeated would grip me and release me, depending on the ebb and flow of anxiety on a given day. But then I would tell myself: this isn't urgent. And as much as I wondered about the bruises themselves, I wondered even more about the energy I was putting into thinking about them. Was this anxiety, or was I tapping into something else? What kind of attention did my worries deserve? There was something more for me to know.

When I finally saw a hematologist, I explained what had been going on. The bruises. The blood test that indicated slow clotting. The hematologist was kind and comforting. He mentioned his adult daughter in passing, and he reminded me of my father. When he asked me questions about my medical history, I could tell that he was listening. He asked me about any tendencies to bleed in excess. I told him I'd been called "a bleeder" when I gave birth. And when he asked if, before the birth of my son, I'd had any prenatal genetic testing done, I told him that I had, and that I'd been told that I was, among other things, a carrier for hemophilia. And it clicked. He suspected that I may in fact have hemophilia. Benevolently excited-seeming, he pointed out that this was "something we only see once every five years or so!" At the end of our conversation, when I told him I had an appointment for a piercing scheduled and asked him if it would be OK for me to go ahead with it before the results of my genetic testing were back, he said "No!" and I felt, amusingly, like I was twelve.

I was, in a matter of a couple of weeks, diagnosed with a mild form of hemophilia. Hemophilia is a rare yet fairly well-known category of genetic blood disorders. It has been mythologized in history and even in popular culture because of its past frequency in royal families, likely beginning with Queen Victoria of England in the nineteenth century (it has at times been referred to as "the royal disease"). Most of all, hemophilia is associated with Tsarevich Alexei of Russia, who suffered so profoundly from bleeding that his mother, the tsarina Alix, sought help from the now-infamous Rasputin. Fundamentally, hemophilia leads to inadequate clotting of the blood, in varying degrees of severity. Hemophilia comes in different forms, depending on deficiencies in different blood proteins known as factors. I soon learned that my case is the result of inadequate factor XI, and as such, is properly known as factor XI deficiency. Symptoms include unexplained bruising.

Upon diagnosis, I felt the best kind of vindication, that rare combination of being, on one hand, right—something was indeed awry—and also, being absolutely fine. My diagnosis is not likely to alter my life in any catastrophic way. I am relieved to have an explanation. Sometimes I ask myself if, after all of this, my life would be meaningfully different had I never received a diagnosis of factor XI deficiency. After all, my case is mild. And I am comforted by my history, comforted by my own body. Before I knew about this diagnosis, I had my wisdom teeth removed, and I was fine. I broke a bone, and I was fine. I got tattoos and piercings. I gave birth. I was fine. So what did I gain in, as is my way, leaving no stone unturned? Practically speaking, knowing matters only in instances of physical trauma. And even then, it is possible that without any special intervention, my blood would clot, and I would be OK. But is it possible that this could one day become vital information? I hope I never find out.

This is an imperfect story, as most true stories are. On one hand, there are meaningful benefits to knowing. Receiving the diagnosis of hemophilia reinstated my confidence in my own sense of my body. My anxiety was my trusty, if vigilant, guide. My worst medical fears were not realized—those are the anxiety at work—but also, I wasn't imagining things. I learned something worth knowing. It wasn't only a diagnosis; it was also a process of finding the space between a feared catastrophe and an instinct rightly followed. In pursuing my questions, I had put my energy somewhere useful. This is anxiety at its best: a survival instinct making itself heard.

But I also know that a better version of these events would have been one in which I could have pursued the same answers without so much struggle, with my energy directed more flexibly. It isn't that I wasn't onto something, that I wasn't rightly insistent—I would do it again. But also, it didn't need to feel so hard. This is the reality— the part that is always a work in progress. You learn, and hopefully it goes a little bit better each time: Anxiety is plastic. It can shape-shift from something dreadful into a new, gentler form, energy for the taking, a force.

The word "hematopoiesis" is, as Dr. Éva Mezey, a scientist who studies stem cells, writes, "a term derived from two Greek words: *haima* (blood) and *poiēsis* (to produce something)." Hematopoietic cells, then, are blood stem cells, meaning that they can become any sort of blood cell. They are plastic in the most extreme sense. Blood within the umbilical cord, known as cord blood, is packed with these hematopoietic cells, and research on cord blood is beginning to untangle the development of a range of diseases, including anxiety disorders.

Studies on cord blood are beginning to demonstrate some of the ways in which maternal mental health may impact changes in fetal DNA and development. In a study on fetal immune system development, researchers found that the cord blood of babies born to mothers experiencing anxiety and stress contained higher levels of cytokines that are associated with problems with the immune system. And in a study on the development of anxiety and depression from birth to early childhood, researchers measured cytokines (essential to immune function and brain development) in cord blood and found lower levels of a particular cytokine known as interleukin 7 (IL-7) in children who later developed symptoms of anxiety and depression. IL-7 is known not only for its influence on brain development but also for reducing inflammation. But as striking as these findings may be, as much as they point toward a connection between the mental health of mothers in pregnancy and their babies' well-being, they are far from conclusive. It is worth noting that in this study, IL-7 was the only cytokine of many that were looked at to be linked to symptoms of anxiety and depression.

Some research suggests that aspects of resilience, too, seem to traverse generations on a biological level. In a recent study, researchers looked at the ways that maternal well-being may be tied to babies' resilience. They found that there was a relationship between maternal resilience as measured in pregnancy and the length of their baby's telomeres at birth. Telomeres, which were measured via cord blood, are a part of our chromosomes that are known to have important implications for psychological health over the course of our lives.

And a study on maternal and fetal levels of brain-derived neuro-trophic factor (BDNF), which plays a crucial role in fetal brain de-velopment, found that during pregnancy, "the placenta provides a barrier protecting the fetus against potentially damaging fluctua-tions in maternal BDNF that occur under conditions of stress." So we see that research on cord blood and mental health is just begin-ning, and it is promising but far from definitive.

Despite these inconclusive research findings, we see, again and again, the incredible plasticity of the body. When a sense like vision is lost, other senses become enhanced. Our blood changes under conditions of stress. We can recover from strokes. And we see that the contents of our blood, our very DNA, is subject to change via forces within and outside ourselves, changes to which we are not fully privy. Where might this plasticity one day lead? What might it make possible? The plasticity of our blood extends into every area of our being—and to our anxiety too. Anxiety, often amorphous, latches on to one thing or another throughout our days and years, whether our health or our work or our personal relationships. It can become anything. It can become panic or paralysis, yet also, it can become a force—the force to complete a task, or the initiative to cre-ate something new, or an urge to connect deeply with someone or see a hidden part of oneself. In this plasticity, there is power.

When you see anxiety in all its malleability, it becomes a force to be channeled. In this way, just as anxiety highlights the precarity of our bodies, it is also a reminder of the stunning flow of life within and around us. When I think about anxiety, I think of the many an-cient principles of our life forces moving through our bodies. I imag-ine my anxiety and my blood together, flowing purposefully through my body, as generative forces of energy and life, instead of sources of dread. I think, too, of humoral theory, in which each of the four bodily humors were associated with a season, and blood aligned with spring. Blood points toward beginnings, but also to endings, loss, and sometimes despair. Blood shows us, with all its paradoxes, how we have no choice but to hold contrasts in our bodies—we are all living alongside the potential for beginnings, and, too, the promise of endings. Anxiety whispers in our ear, insistently: *Is this the beginning? Is this the end?* But really, the two are not so far apart. It is the beginning. It is the end. So much is possible. Blood, and anxiety, tells us this too.

Part III

HEART

REGULATION AND PERSEVERANCE

More than anything, the heart wants to beat.

—Sandeep Jauhar, *Heart: A History*

Long before medicine as we now know it, it was the heart, rather than the brain, that was believed to be the seat of thought. In ancient Egypt, the heart was understood to be a place of intellect, emotion, and wisdom. Aristotle believed that thinking originated in the heart. Notably, though, in the Hippocratic Corpus, which dates back to the fifth century BCE, Hippocrates (or, potentially, his contemporaries) wrote, "Some say too that we think with our hearts and it is the heart which suffers pain and feels anxiety. There is no truth in this." These functions were instead attributed to the brain. Nonetheless, in the eleventh century, Avicenna, a Persian philosopher and medical practitioner, argued that the heart orchestrated the functioning of the rest of the body. But before we understood the precise functioning of the heart in the body, we knew, on a visceral level, that there is a thread that links our hearts to our psychology. In the early seventeenth century, describing melancholy (which, you will recall, at the time encompassed what we now term anxiety disorders), Robert Burton described changes in heart rate as a consequence of anxiety: "Some add palpitations of the heart, cold sweat, as usual Symptoms, and a leaping in many parts of the body." A leaping! Our understanding of the heart has changed, but its centrality in our conceptions of our bodies and minds remains. Through ever-evolving research, we are coming to see how it is that the heart communicates with the entirety of the body and even with forces outside of ourselves, and in so doing, shapes our well-being.

For all its complexity, most of the time the heart doesn't feel particularly abstract. It is a constant, seemingly knowable part of our everyday lives. We know that our hearts behave differently under different conditions. I know, for instance, that my heart rate will increase when I exercise. I know that when I feel, to varying degrees, fearful or anxious or embarrassed or even excited, my heart beats especially quickly. I know, too, a certain sense of breathlessness, of my heart accelerating, in moments of overwhelming joy—my heart seems to "skip a beat." It is common knowledge that the heart and the brain are interacting in these moments—that there is a link between the way we feel and the ways in which our hearts function—yet this interaction is, for most of us, poorly understood. As a psychologist, I've thought a great deal about the ways anxiety can manifest in the heart, both in my clinical work and in myself—yet many of the available explanations are unsatisfying or incomplete. As tends to be the case, the more we learn about the complex interactions between our hearts and our emotional lives, we see that there is much we don't know—much that remains open to scientific inquiry, and, too, aspects of the heart that resist science altogether.

Anxiety manifests in the heart with particular force, sometimes long before we know precisely what it is that is troubling us. The James-Lange theory of emotion, which was developed in the late nineteenth century, argued that before we have feelings (like anxiety), we have bodily sensations—and that it is those sensations that tell us something about how we are feeling. Within this framework, physical sensations precede thoughts. When it comes to the brain and the heart, we ask: What happens first? Do we feel the beating of our hearts accelerate and then come to a thought (say, "I'm anxious!"), or do anxious thoughts give rise to an increase in heart rate? A bodily sensation and then a state of mind? Or a state of mind and then a bodily sensation?

When our hearts respond to anxiety, they demand urgent action. People in the midst of panic attacks often fear that they are, in that moment, dying of a heart attack, or otherwise, that they are losing their mind. (In fact, among the DSM 5 criteria for panic disorder are "fear of dying" and "fear of losing control or 'going crazy.'") These symptoms are commonly reported in psychotherapy—and they can be terrifying, so much so that they are often the reason that a person decides to begin treatment. The urgent can, as is said, overtake the important, and to work through anxiety, we need to learn to recognize the difference. What feels momentarily like imminent cardiac danger can overshadow the underlying factors that actually shape and perpetuate anxiety. When our hearts overwhelm us, when they seem to beat out of control, they make our fears concrete. They insist that we pay attention. In the moment, the fear is something like, "Am I having a heart attack in this instant?" We feel a sense of imminent threat rather than the low thrum of existential dread.

When I began having panic attacks as a teenager, which invariably included a racing heart, I, like so many people with anxiety, initially believed that the problem I had was cardiac in nature. Even after I learned that that wasn't the case, I continued to attempt to take apart the panic attacks, looking for explanations for my distress within the structure and functioning of my heart. Though I couldn't fully articulate it at the time, I know now that I was looking for a bodily solution, one that I hoped would be more straightforward than the tumult of my mind.

Things were different then, and then was not so long ago. At the time, to attribute what was happening in my body to anxiety felt shameful and weak. I hadn't, in any direct sense, been made to feel this way by others—on the contrary, my family was, and continues to be, especially empathic to the ways of anxiety. Nonetheless, I was, as we all are, subject to long-standing cultural forces that view anxiety as a personal shortcoming. In my small hometown, therapy was something to whisper about, more a last resort than a lifestyle. Anxiety wasn't a point of conversation in my social circle, even among my closest friends, at least not in any direct sense. We talked about all sorts of intimate matters, had known each other since elementary school, but anxiety was left largely unnamed and unspoken. Years later, well into adulthood, I learned that some of my closest friends had had similar struggles. I imagine the conversations we could have had, had we realized the camaraderie that was, in fact, within our reach.

It's not unusual to initially conceptualize anxiety as a purely physical process. People struggling with anxiety may avoid activities that increase their heart rate (for instance, taking the elevator rather than the stairs or no longer exercising) because the physical sensations of their heart rate increasing can evoke panic. People often come to psychotherapy with bodily symptoms that their doctors have not found a physical explanation for—symptoms like a racing heart or a tight feeling in the chest. To be fair, it's not unreasonable to be frightened by these symptoms, as they are in fact the body's alarm system in action and they can be symptoms of heart problems. Internet lists of strategies for distinguishing a panic attack from a heart attack are wildly unsatisfying—especially when you are panicked. But even after the initial relief of ruling out cardiac explanations, the anxiety soon returns.

Unlike most of our organs, we are able to feel our hearts beating, even when we are well—whereas the functioning of most of our organs, like, say, the liver, is opaque to us without medical intervention. People are aware of the beating of their hearts to varying degrees—some of us notice and pay attention to them often, whereas others only tune in to their rhythms when they are especially rapid or otherwise out of the ordinary—during cardiovascular exercise, say, or in times of fear or anxiety. Awareness of one's own internal bodily sensations—from, for instance, a momentary wave of nausea to a tickle in the throat or a subtle shift in heart rate—is a phenomenon known as interoception. The heart can be the focus of a great deal of interoceptive experience. We feel shifts in our heart rate throughout the day, many of which (but, importantly, not necessarily all) are part of the ordinary functioning of the body. But also, our hearts provide

131

a direct, sensory link to the aliveness of our bodies, and especially so when we are anxious. They remind us of our fragility as human beings—that we have bodies upon which we are utterly dependent.

Anxiety disorders are often associated with higher levels of interoception. There is a degree of safety in noticing changes in the body—it leads us to get necessary medical care more quickly—but heightened interoception can become a problem when it turns the corner toward hypervigilance. For this reason, high levels of interoception tend to be framed as an obstacle in the context of anxiety disorders.

But this dynamic isn't straightforward. Interoception encompasses multiple facets, including interoceptive accuracy and interoceptive awareness. It is one thing to be correct in your interpretation of bodily sensations and another to be paying attention to them. A recent meta-analysis found no relationship between accurate cardiac interoception and anxiety. That is, across many studies, there was no indication that anxious people were especially *accurate* when asked to, for instance, count their own heartbeats over a period of time. In thinking through their results, the researchers point out that perhaps it isn't increased interoceptive accuracy that heightens anxiety, but rather the degree of attention to one's own internal state that does so. I've seen many times the ways in which heightened interoception (even if inaccurate) exacerbates panic and anxiety more broadly. Sensations that are simply the normal functioning of the body—like, say, a grumbling in the stomach or a cramp in one's side—are easily misinterpreted as harmful.

When we learn that anxiety and its accompanying bodily sensations will not overtake us, anxiety beings to lose its grip. Little by little, space emerges to work through the internal struggles that have been relegated to the body, and which often manifest physically in the heart. Across psychotherapeutic modalities, interventions to counter symptoms of anxiety often work via the body, with common practices including breathing techniques and progressive muscle relaxation. These physical processes can, over time, reduce bodily hyperactivation, slow the breath, and with it, the heart rate, and bring about a state of bodily calm. They are some among many of the practices that fall under the umbrella of "distress tolerance" skills.

In an extensive review of research on distress tolerance, distress tolerance is defined as both "the *perceived* capacity to withstand negative emotional and/or other aversive states elicited by some type of stressor" and "the *behavioral act* of withstanding distressing internal states elicited by some type of stressor." In recent decades, the term "distress tolerance" has become part of the therapeutic vernacular to describe strategies that we use to soothe ourselves when we are struggling, and more broadly, to describe one's capacity to move through emotional pain. In keeping with the formal definitions, "perception" and "withstanding" are central. When we perceive ourselves as able to weather a difficult period of time, rather than perceiving ourselves as ill-equipped to do so, this shapes our emotional state and our behavior. And when we think about anxiety (and other difficult emotional states) as something we can withstand, rather than feelings to be banished, we expand our capacity for resilience.

Distress tolerance skills are most often attributed to dialectical behavior therapy (DBT), a form of therapy that was created by psychologist Marsha Linehan. Though Linehan is most famous for her pioneering work in developing a treatment for borderline personality disorder, her approach is powerful across a number of other diagnoses, and distress tolerance skills drawing from DBT can be helpful for anxiety symptoms. Distress tolerance skills are wide-ranging, and sometimes they act directly on the body. The acronym TIPP is used to refer to "temperature, intense exercise, paced breathing, paired muscle relaxation." These are skills that people employ to respond to an intense, upsetting emotion—like anxiety. Imagine a person who feels overcome by panic. Their heart is racing, they are sweating, they feel utterly overwhelmed, they begin to cry, and then they become afraid that they are going to hyperventilate. According to TIPP, they might put their face in a bowl of ice cold water, thus lowering their heart rate, or do thirty jumping jacks to expend energy, or practice five minutes of diaphragmatic breathing. These strategies have direct impact on the body and on cardiac functioning in particular. By shifting the way that your body feels, distress tolerance skills help drain off the intense physical discomfort of anxiety, and then, they create a sense of capability—of experiencing your own capacity to shift your state of mind. They can be a way forward, to the next moment and the next and the next—a guide to perseverance, and, eventually, resilience.

Researchers are homing in on the role of distress tolerance in treating anxiety. People who are high in distress tolerance (meaning that they bear their distress well) seem to be less sensitive to anxiety and more tolerant of uncertainty than those who are low in distress tolerance. Indeed, distress tolerance is negatively associated with anxiety and OCD symptoms—which is to say that people with symptoms of anxiety and OCD may have lower levels of distress tolerance. But no matter where your starting point is, distress tolerance is something you can cultivate. Among other things, mindfulness seems to be helpful in developing greater distress tolerance and may, in this way, help to reduce symptoms of anxiety and depression.

Daniel Siegel, a psychiatrist who, you will recall, is also an expert on mindfulness, coined the term "window of tolerance" in the late 1990s. He writes, "Each of us has a 'window of tolerance' in which various intensities of emotional arousal can be processed without disrupting the functioning of the system." When it comes to expanding one's window of tolerance, mindfulness practices (like meditation) can be powerful because they encourage us to observe and tolerate difficult emotions rather than attempting to resolve them or push them away. The "window of tolerance" has become a highly influential framework for thinking about our responses to trauma and to other forms of stress. Elizabeth Stanley, PhD, an expert on recovery from trauma and stress, writes, "our neurobiological *window of tolerance* to stress arousal is *the window within which we are capable of adjusting our stress levels upward or downward to remain, over time, within the optimal performance zone of moderate arousal.*" Fundamentally, resilience comes down to our capacity for adjustment, for flexibility. When we are resilient, we are able to live well without too much interruption, even when under stress. It follows that in many ways, resilience hinges on cultivating a wider window of tolerance to discomfort and to hard times.

We are all looking for ways to soothe ourselves—but no matter the forms of distress tolerance you use, they require regular practice. Anxiety comes and goes, and like most things in life, relief wears off. By learning to introduce a sense of calm at a physical level, you can begin to go further, to explore what is driving your anxiety. What meaning might I attribute to the acceleration of my heart, the tightening in my chest, in this moment? Knowing that I can withstand this moment, knowing that this moment will pass, how can I turn these bodily sensations into understanding? In this way, distress tolerance practices build upon themselves, into a kind of strength.

Research continues to support our intuitive understanding that anxiety and the heart are in constant conversation. It follows, then, that if we pay attention to anxiety when it emerges, it may be possible to intervene in ways that change the course of anxiety and of cardiac health too.

Biofeedback training is a therapeutic method that is sometimes used for the treatment of anxiety disorders, and which is generally supported by research. The goal of this treatment is to reduce anxiety by using data about patients' own bodies alongside anxiety-reduction techniques. They make changes in the body measurable, concrete, and there can be a degree of instant gratification. So, for instance, a patient diagnosed with panic disorder might wear a heart-rate sensor during a psychotherapy session in which panic is deliberately evoked, practice diaphragmatic breathing during the session, and then observe, on the sensor, the corresponding reduction in their heart rate. For some people, this experience is empowering. They see that their deliberate, paced breathing made a quantifiable change in their body, and they feel their anxiety recede. For others, it feels like a statement of the obvious and has little bearing on the recurrence of their anxiety symptoms. Biofeedback training is, as the name suggests, a sort of teaching tool—it aims to teach patients about the ways their bodies respond to different experiences, and that as such, their bodies are capable of responding positively to therapeutic interventions too. But also, it is a treatment that demonstrates, in concrete terms, our capacity to foster a sort of interorgan communication.

Even without formal monitoring, our bodies are constantly giving us feedback, much of which passes us by in the course of the day. When you exercise, especially on days when you would rather not, you will often find that afterward there is an improvement in your mood and energy level. This is feedback, and ideally you make a mental note of it and it helps you to exercise again the next day. Certainly, when we eat, we receive feedback—our bodies feel, perhaps, energized, sated . . . or they don't. And when it comes to anxiety, we are capable of making similar observations. One might, for instance, notice physical sensations of anxiety emerging during a work meeting, and then use a breathing technique for a few minutes and note that their palms stop sweating and their heart rate slows.

The visceral experience of anxiety in the heart is only the beginning (or, really, the middle). In fact, research suggests that anxiety can have a lasting impact on cardiac well-being. Anxiety and obsessive-compulsive disorder are now being linked, through empirical research, to a range of forms of cardiovascular disease. On one hand, these findings are intuitive—we've known, for much of human history, that our bodies and our emotional states are linked, long before we had hard data to support this experience. During periods of anxiety, we feel the manifestation of physical tension just as we feel our heart rate increase. Yet we remain accustomed to, and even comforted by, writing off these bodily shifts as trivial and unworthy of our attention—as "just anxiety." Research suggests that this is misguided.

Anxiety and hypertension often co-occur. In a large meta-analysis (one that included data from over four million participants), researchers identified a significant link between anxiety and hypertension—in fact, they go so far as to point out that "longitudinal data and theoretical literature indicate that anxiety may *precede* hypertension." This is remarkable because it suggests that anxiety may sometimes *cause* hypertension. Another team of researchers found that it is anxiety in particular that links high emotional reactivity (briefly put, having intense, overwhelming, long-lasting reactions) to increases in blood pressure. That is, when they examined the link between emotional reactivity and high blood pressure, it turned out that anxiety actually explained their connection. Research in this vein points toward enormous potential when it comes to the treatment and prevention of anxiety, if only we pay attention to it. Treating anxiety as something real—something worth working through, rather than something to brush off—may bring about life-changing improvements in health.

Though we tend to think of our hearts beating evenly when we are calm, in fact, ideally, there is variation (inconsistencies that are too small for us to feel) in our heart rate. This is known as heart rate variability, or HRV. Healthy HRV indicates that our hearts can function flexibly, whereas low HRV (too little variation) is associated with a higher risk of cardiac problems, and, too, with anxiety disorders. We seem to benefit from flexibility across domains—the cardiac rigidity associated with low HRV mirrors the emotional rigidity that anxiety brings about.

There is no avoiding the constant interplay between our emotional and physical experiences. Even as I write this sentence, I'm struck by the ways that using two separate terms for these dimensions of human life is not quite right, that words fail me. Too often, the emotional and the physical become linked to that which is concrete (the body) and that which isn't (the mind). As the empirical evidence mounts demonstrating the constant interaction between our emotional and physical lives, psychology and psychiatry are facing difficult questions about the ways we think about concrete, numbers-based interventions and the more elusive yet nonetheless profound shifts that can happen within us. How far does understanding our biology, our physiology, take us when it comes to anxiety? And then, how far can insight about our own histories and present struggles take us? To move forward, we need ideas, and science, that can do both.

In 1994, Stephen Porges, PhD, introduced the polyvagal theory at a conference on psychophysiology research. The following year, he published a now seminal paper on his theory that has come to shape the field of trauma research and has had massive impact on the field of psychology more broadly. Porges writes that "when humans feel safe, their nervous systems support the homeostatic functions of health, growth, and restoration, while they simultaneously become accessible to others without feeling or expressing threat and vulnerability," and as such, he refers to polyvagal theory as "a science of safety."

With polyvagal theory, Porges takes on the physiology of feeling safe, and the ways in which our hearts and our central nervous systems interact when we feel safe, or, conversely, when we feel threatened or afraid. Polyvagal theory is big—it traverses the body, linking the heart and the brain, the nervous system more broadly, the lungs, and even the muscles of the face. The vagus is a cranial nerve, meaning it begins in the brain, and the term "polyvagal" refers to the fact that in mammals, the vagal nerve has two branches, which are associated with different functions. Porges explains that "the polyvagal theory . . . provides an explanation of how the vagal pathways regulate heart rate in response to novelty and to a variety of stressors." According to polyvagal theory, our responses to new situations and information are shaped by the vagus and fall under three categories: immobilization—when we shut down, often in traumatic circumstances; mobilization, which is the classic fight-or-flight response; and social engagement, which is our ideal state of being, one in which we feel safe and can connect meaningfully with others.

Polyvagal theory has recently moved into the mainstream, even becoming a fixture on TikTok. Influencers describe attempting to, for instance, "tune" their vagal nerve to reduce anxiety. I spoke to Porges about his work (which, as we know, has been ongoing for decades) and asked him what he thinks of its newfound place in popular culture. He told me that most of all, he wants it to be known that "it's not that you hack your nervous system." No, there are no hacks. There are, however, a number of clinicians who are developing sophisticated therapeutic techniques to treat physiological responses to trauma and anxiety, as well as conditions like autism, through the lens of polyvagal theory. Fundamentally, these polyvagal approaches to psychotherapy are geared toward helping people to experience states of safety, and then connection.

Though polyvagal theory tends to be discussed with respect to trauma, it is also hugely useful in thinking about anxiety—because anxiety and trauma can evoke similar physiological responses. In both cases, there is a profound, bodily felt sense of feeling threatened or unsafe. When I spoke to Porges, I asked him how he thinks of polyvagal theory with respect to anxiety in particular. He told me, "I think anxiety is a bad word." That is, he sees anxiety as a physiological state. Talking with him, I'm struck by his ability to see human behavior in physical terms—to think of anxiety as knowable, identifiable through measures of heart rate or sweating, for instance—but simultaneously in profoundly human, empathic terms. Central to polyvagal theory is the principle of co-regulation. Porges sees feelings of safety as emerging out of social experiences rather than something that occurs when we are in isolation. These social experiences begin at birth between a newborn and their mother, and if we are lucky, they shape our lives and foster a sense of being safe in the world. A felt sense of safety can emerge in conversation with a trusted teacher, or by spending time with a close friend, or in the comfort of reciprocal love. And though one could argue that these are in many respects physiological experiences, they are also something else, something that measurement can't touch. Soon after speaking with him, I attend a talk at a trauma conference where Porges describes co-regulation ever so poignantly, saying, "The nervous system has to be convinced it's not alone."

&

It's tempting to think of the heart as, ultimately, a pump—just a machine. In recent decades, we've taken many steps forward thanks to research on the role of the heart in our emotional well-being. We see, through the lens of science, the ways in which our feelings and our bodies are in constant conversation with each other. Yet despite all that we are learning about the workings of the heart, we are reminded that there remains much we don't understand, much that eludes science altogether. The heart remains a place whose meaning extends far beyond its mechanistic role in the body. In this way, the heart pushes the envelope on questions central to mental health today: To what degree are mental health and physical health equivalent? How can we come to understand the relationship between the body and the mind? And can they be understood through the same paradigms?

These are age-old problems. We seem to wrestle endlessly with the place of the body and the mind and how it is that the two meet, and we have yet to arrive at satisfying answers. And lest we go so far as to think that we're now coming to some new level of higher awareness, history shows us otherwise. Nearly a century ago, in 1928, Carl Jung wrote, "The fascination of the psyche brings about a new self-appraisal, a reassessment of our fundamental human nature. We can hardly be surprised if this leads to a rediscovery of the body after its long subjection to the spirit—we are even tempted to say that the flesh is getting its own back." Reading Jung today, I'm reminded that it isn't only that the body and mind are inseparable, though that is fundamentally true, but that to ignore the body is to ignore a piece of our humanness. When it comes to anxiety, the flesh is indeed getting its own back. Our heart, with all of its sensations, remains our most direct link to the aliveness of our body. We feel it beating, and we feel its rhythms reflecting our innermost states, for better and for worse. In this way, the heart is a constant reminder of the uncertainty of our bodies, and of life itself—and, too, of what it is to be alive. We feel our heart pumping, we feel the persistence of the body day in and day out, and we remember that we are here, in this moment, in the flesh, undeniably. That when it comes to the mind and to the body, we must be humble. That there is much we don't know. There are some questions without answers, and it is for us to learn to live with the questions. But how alive we are!

In ancient Egypt, it was believed that when a person died, their body should be preserved—mummified—so that their spirit would be able to find it in the afterlife. Mummification prevented the spirit from getting lost. And in early periods of Egyptian history, when bodies were prepared for mummification, all the internal organs were removed, except for the heart. Even in death, the heart was indispensable.

This is the story of the Egyptian sun god, Re:

> In the morning he was Khepri—the scarab beetle—slowly rolling the great ball of the sun above the horizon; at midday he was Re, the most powerful manifestation of the sun god; and in the evening, he was the weary ram-headed Atum . . . ready to be reenergized for the coming morning.

It is in this way that the scarab beetle came to symbolize regeneration and rebirth. Amulets in the form of heart scarabs were sometimes placed with the dead, with an inscription, known as the heart scarab spell, that began: "My heart, my mother; my heart, my mother! My heart whereby I came into being!" We remember our aliveness and our capacity for perseverance. Tomorrow is a new day.

6.

ANCHORS: STORY, LOVE, AND BELONGING

> In Orphism Eros is regarded as the creator
> god. . . . He is the god of beginnings, or origins,
> of the possibility of new beginnings.
>
> —Christine Downing, "Towards an
> Erotics of the Psyche"

A long time ago, science and art were not so far apart. To study the heavens, the earth, and the body was to be in conversation with art, literature, and even theology. Mystery abounded, and with so much yet to be discovered, the divide between science and art was elastic. The thread of reverence that runs through all kinds of learning was strong, and there was room for wonder and pragmatism to coexist.

Today, we are reaping the benefits of recent centuries' advances in the study of the heart—how our hearts work, and why, sometimes, they don't. We know that our heart rate is linked to our emotional state, and that it increases when we are anxious. Our blood pressure too. We even know that cardiac health can deteriorate in the context of chronic anxiety. And we've seen, too, that anxiety accumulates in our bodies, in our hearts, in ways that we aren't always aware of. But as it turns out, the old philosophers weren't all wrong. Although our understandings of the heart have evolved dramatically over time, and we no longer see it as the organ of thought that it was once believed to be, the heart remains a powerful symbol of feeling, of love, and of connection. Our hearts seem to swell with joy. They feel as though they could burst out of our chests with pride or break when love is lost. In the midst of scientific advancement, we run the risk of losing sight of the other meanings that our hearts convey.

The symbolism of the heart reminds us that psychology and psychiatry, neuroscience and biology, leave some of our most deeply felt anxieties unspoken for. That there are parts of life—some beautiful and others horrific—for which we have no complete explanation. I am, most sincerely, eternally grateful for the ways that we use these fields of understanding to ease anxiety. But I also know that some of the most powerful antidotes available to us lie far outside the world of psychopharmacology, and outside the consulting room too. Without another kind of heart, we lose contact with fundamental aspects of our humanity. The heart is what we know it to be—an organ pumping blood—yet it stands for far more. It always has, and it always will. In the heart, we find the wisdom of people before us and hope for those who will follow us. We see that although there is no cure for anxiety, although there are some anxieties that we will carry with us forever, in the carrying, we are never really alone.

How do we move through periods of anxiety that seem to capture our attention and our bodies in their entirety? We know that we can use techniques like, say, diaphragmatic breathing or progressive muscle relaxation to begin to regulate our hearts. But this is only the beginning. When I feel anxiety creeping in, I try to align myself with a sense of the world that is far bigger than my own experience—one where I can see my anxiety gaining form and meaning, by drawing upon wisdom outside myself. Of course, this is one thing to say and another thing altogether to do. It feels like tuning my ear to a language I used to know. Far off at first, hard to grasp—and then deeply familiar, part of myself, sometimes dormant but always there. Story. Love. Togetherness. They are age-old responses to anxiety—they reflect the humanity at the very center of it—and they are the threads that bond us.

We come to the ways that the heart and its relationship to anxiety teach us about the most powerful aspects of our emotional lives: the stories we live by, and the relationships that are most essential to our lives. The intertwining of story and human connection is at the heart of our very existence, it forms our humanity.

Anxiety emerges with particular force when life feels chaotic, and we know that people who experience significant anxiety are especially sensitive to uncertainty. Over the course of our lives, chaos and uncertainty seem to emerge and recede, depending on our dispositions and our experiences. Stories have always been a response to chaos—they bring form and meaning to our amorphous distress. Through the stories that we share with one another, we face those unanswerable, eternally relevant questions—and we see that our struggles to accept the limits and the uncertainty of our lives are nothing new, and that they are part of what makes us human.

Mythologies from around the world show us life emerging out of chaos. We've always seemed to see ourselves through this sort of story, in which form comes from what seemed formless. The myth of P'an Ku, from Chinese mythology, tells us: "At first there was nothing. Time passed and nothing became something." In Quiché Mayan mythology, the story goes: "Thus let it be done! Let the emptiness be filled! Let the water recede and make a void, let the earth appear and become solid; let it be done." And from Greek and Roman mythology, "At first all was chaos. . . . Chaos was infinite and dark, a yawning chasm through which the jumbled elements that make up the world were forever falling." In each of these stories, we learn about an empty, uncertain beginning. Over and over, we fill the void. Stories tell us something about where we came from and where we might be going. That we aren't in free fall. They say, *You weren't the first, nor are you alone*, and they say, *This means something.*

And stories have always played a part in teaching us about the limits of our control and understanding. In ancient Greek literature, where fate had a heavy hand in the course of people's lives, stories were determined in advance. In *The Iliad*, consumed with grief and rage, Hecuba says to Priam:

> We sit here in our great hall far away,
>
> mourning our son, for whom strong Destiny
>
> assigned this ending when she spun his thread,
>
> when he was born, when I gave birth to him—
>
> that he would fall beneath some forceful man
>
> and glut the hunger of the swift-pawed dogs

far from his parents. I wish I could latch

my teeth into the center of his liver

and eat it!

Hecuba and Priam's catastrophe had been predetermined. It was no less tragic, no less devastating—but it was out of mortal hands.

On an individual scale, we have our own stories, our own myths. Anxiety can generate its own pernicious mythmaking. These are another kind of stories of catastrophe told in advance—of the awful things that could be, instead of what already is. I recall a wise psychologist who described anxiety, aptly, as "the tyranny of what-ifs." But then, we are capable of a subtle but essential shift—we can tell generative stories, too, of beginnings and endings, of joy, and of loss. Most of all, we tell stories—and seek out the stories of others—about the things that trouble us. When I read stories about terminally ill teenagers as a child, I see now that I was beginning to face my anxiety about mortality. In my twenties, when I, stubbornly faithless, read books and watched reality TV about Mormonism (like *Under the Banner of Heaven* by Jon Krakauer, and then and, I admit, still, *Sister Wives* on TLC), I think I was trying to understand the ways that some people's anxiety responds to faith—and where my own skepticism meets my wish for assurance. When we look back on the stories that most engage us, whether in books or elsewhere, we can find a sort of post-hoc biography of our anxieties. The stories that we encounter, and then, the ones that we tell about ourselves, shape our sense of identity. They inform what we feel capable of and what feels impossible. And anxiety influences these narratives at every turn.

Will I allow my fear to drive my decisions? What could be lost, but also, what could be? It is not lost on me that writing this book is, for me, a way to construct a story of anxiety, a narrative with shape and direction and purpose.

Whether they are articulated in art or in the context of psychotherapy, stories show us ourselves, and more, and in this way, they take us beyond ourselves. Stories are a chance to find language for, or put language to, our anxieties. In an essay on the relationship between psychoanalysis and poetry, psychoanalyst and writer Adam Phillips says, "One goes to psychoanalysis, as one might go to poetry, for better words." With the right words, the right story, we get to the heart of things, and in this way, there is twofold relief: the relief in hearing something true, and also the relief in doing so with another person, both a partner and a witness. Through the stories of our lives, we give form and meaning to experiences we previously struggled to articulate.

In literature, poetry, film, and other forms of art, stories can contain a psychological sophistication that simply isn't subject to theoretical models or statistics. In the words of literary critic Lionel Trilling, "To pass from the reading of a great literary work to a treatise of academic psychology is to pass from one order of perception to another." Although science will never, I believe, fully capture the power that stories contain, empirical research is beginning to demonstrate their benefits for the body. A recent study found that among children who were hospitalized in the intensive care unit, after being told a story, there was a decrease in their cortisol levels (a hormone associated with stress), a rise in their oxytocin levels (a hormone associated with lower levels of stress), and a reduction in pain. Research has also, for decades, demonstrated the importance of imaginative play for children. When children play, they construct narratives, they tell stories to themselves and to one another. This is a natural, necessary form of working things through, trying to understand the world, to harness a sense of power when they have little of it.

My son, like many children, loves to hear the story of his birth. I remember writing notes to myself on the first few days after he was born, wanting to be sure that I wouldn't forget the details. But the story I tell him now is a different version altogether. It leaves out much of what I wrote down, details that seem mostly arbitrary to me now, like what time contractions began and how dilated my cervix was when we arrived at the hospital. This story is for him. It is a story of his beginning. Each time I tell him this story, he hears that we were waiting, so eagerly, for his arrival. That he was ready to be born, squished inside, and grouchy on arrival, that we loved his grouchiness—that we loved him before he was born. This story forms a groundwork for him, a sense of love that preceded his birth, a love that he will always have within him. In this story, one body emerges from another one, and for a while, anything feels possible.

But there can be too much of a good thing. When the stories that we hear and tell about ourselves become rigid, they can create new problems. In *Strangers to Ourselves*, journalist Rachel Aviv explores the ways in which our stories can become limiting factors in the sphere of mental health. She writes, "Mental illnesses are often seen as chronic and intractable forces that take over our lives, but I wonder how much the stories we tell about them, especially in the beginning, can shape their course. People can feel freed by these stories, but they can also get stuck in them." When anxiety becomes the overwhelming narrative of one's life, when the story loses its elasticity, it doesn't frame or expand so much as it confines. Anxiety (or other sorts of struggles) can become a fallback explanation, a heuristic that conceals other factors at play.

I treated a patient who, like many people do, came to treatment for anxiety. She couldn't sleep and had begun to worry far more than usual about small decisions. She described feeling jittery and irritable much of the time. She knew anxiety well—she had struggled with it since childhood. Her anxiety would come and go depending on her circumstances, and she had been in and out of treatment for a decade or so. At the start of treatment, she told me that she knew she was an anxious person, that she always had been and always would be. What she was after in treatment were strategies to help her with her insomnia and to feel less irritable with her fiancé.

Ideally, therapy helps us to see the blind spots in our narratives. As treatment unfolded, we came to address her feelings of dissatisfaction in areas of her life that she saw as fait accompli. And little by little, she expressed ambivalence about central areas of her life—like her long-standing engagement and her professional trajectory. Her anxiety was, as always, a symptom, and as she developed greater clarity around her uncertainties, her initial symptoms began to resolve. When you stop at a word, at a title, a diagnosis, you miss opportunities for exploration and change.

We discover the stories of our lives as we articulate them over time—and they evolve. I've found that people who come to move through anxiety with a sense of depth and even grace seem to create a flexible narrative of themselves and their lives, chaos and all. They see strength in forming an internal story that evolves over time, and they find reason to be interested in the process. They don't hold themselves at arm's length—it isn't a matter of distance or abstraction. They live through pain as we all must—but rather than a cross to bear, their story becomes an ongoing conversation, between words and the body, the body and words, and back again. This perpetual translation isn't a straightforward, one-to-one equation. There are gains and there are losses. It isn't as simple as: my racing heart is my anxiety, or, my anxiety explains all my experiences. Instead, there is a constant interplay among our physiology and our emotions and the stories we believe about ourselves. In this way, the stories of our lives unfold, and their meaning expands and reshapes itself. Indeed, love and change and our most closely held stories have always been intertwined. In his work on Greek and Roman mythology, Philip Matyszak writes, "The primeval Eros was a mighty force . . . for without Eros the other beings who sprang from Chaos would have remained static and unchanging, eternal yet sterile. For Eros embodied not only love but also the entire reproductive principle. . . . The universe of myth was created through love."

As a teenager, I became briefly fascinated with images of hearts. But somehow, even while writing about the heart, I had forgotten about this period in my life. And then, while going through old photographs in my father's attic, I found boxes of my childhood belongings. Amid the journals and CDs and crystals, I found collages of hearts, homemade books with heart bindings, even a bag I had knit in the shape of a heart. These objects date back to when I first had a panic attack and thus became, for a time, concerned about the state of my own heart.

Then, when I was seventeen, I secretly got a tattoo. It was an asymmetrical, wobbly-looking heart that I'd drawn. The tattoo artist asked if I wanted the asymmetry corrected and I said no—this was my way of conveying my sense of feeling, of the imperfection of our hearts and minds, made literal. My best friends came with me, and we were all thrilled by the rebellion. But I couldn't keep the secret—within a few days, I confessed what I'd done to my parents, and the way that I built up what I was about to tell them, they were relieved that it was only a tattoo. I wouldn't feel compelled to get the same tattoo today, but I don't mind it. It means something else to me now. I see with greater clarity the layers of meaning that were unfolding. It was, for me, a feeling, an emerging identity, and a small rebellion, embodied. It tells a different story now.

 ↶

In love, in all of its many forms, we experience those most beautiful moments in life—true connection, mutual reverence, and intimacy—despite life's uncertainties and despite the losses that we all inevitably endure. Whether between parent and child, in friendship, in romantic relationships, or in that expansive sort of love that extends beyond our own circles and evokes a larger human bond, love of all sorts ties us together. Of all the heart's symbolic meanings, it is love that we hear about most of all, so much so that it runs the risk of being overwrought. But the symbol sticks for good reason.

Research suggests that love and social bonding impact the ways in which stress and anxiety manifest in our life experiences and in our bodies in profound ways, and we see these effects across the lifespan.

In a recent study on the physiological impact of hugs between babies and parents, researchers found that as early as about four months of age, babies experience changes in heart rate that indicate reduced stress when being hugged by their parents, more so than when being hugged by a stranger. And they found that parents' heart rates also change to indicate reduced stress when hugging their baby. There are measurable, positive changes in our bodies in response to this exchange of love.

Into adulthood, bodily responses to stress remain connected to experiences of love. In a study that compared the physiological responses of single adults and newly coupled adults to movies with content described as "positive" or "negative," researchers found greater indications of bodily stress in the singles group. They argue that "love and attachment [may] provide a buffer against the experience of stress." The anxiolytic (anxiety-reducing) properties of relationships seem to extend into the realm of friendship too. In a meta-analysis, researchers found that for adolescents, "positive peer relationships" may play a protective role when it comes to social anxiety. And a study on older adults' well-being found that those who experienced more compassionate love, which includes love in a broad context of relationships, reported lower symptoms of anxiety—and this link was explained by the fact that compassionate love reduced loneliness, in turn reducing anxiety.

We find again and again that though certain kinds of relationships and interpersonal experiences can help to protect us against anxiety, anxiety can also impact the formation of relationships. People who experience social anxiety often struggle with dating and with intimacy in romantic relationships. We see, too, that anxiety at a young age may have implications for future relationships. A recent study linked children's behavior in early adolescence to their relationship status decades later. Researchers found that children who were observed to be anxious were more likely to be single as adults, or to become partnered later in adulthood, than others. Another study looked at the ways in which people with anxiety disorders relate to criticism in romantic relationships. They found that "compared to individuals without psychopathology, individuals with anxiety disorders perceive their partners to be more critical of them" and also that "individuals with anxiety disorders are more critical of their romantic partners when discussing a problem topic." Across the lifespan, anxiety and trouble with relationships can form a vicious, self-reinforcing cycle. The relationships in our lives that provide real connection (and, presumably, those that reduce anxiety levels) are those in which we can feel, quite simply, at ease within ourselves, and that ease can be elusive. It's often said that an ounce of prevention is worth a pound of cure, and when it comes to anxiety and relationships, this is surely true.

Loneliness is consistently shown to have massive implications for our health, mental and otherwise, and it is consistently associated with both depression and anxiety. A recent study looked at experiences of loneliness, the relative presence of social networks, and symptoms of depression and anxiety in adults fifty and older. By measuring these dimensions at two points in time with two years between them, researchers found that there was a two-way street between loneliness and symptoms of anxiety, meaning each may perpetuate the other.

Research links loneliness to other forms of disease too. In a powerful paper on the problems of loneliness for our well-being, Minhal

Ahmed, Ivo Cerda, and Molly Maloof frame loneliness as a kind of stress on the body, one that can have major implications for our health. They point to the work of the late John Cacioppo, PhD, one of the world's foremost scholars on loneliness, who wrote, along with William Patrick, "Loneliness not only alters behavior but shows up in measurements of stress hormones, immune function, and cardiovascular function. Over time, these changes in physiology are compounded in ways that may be hastening millions of people to an early grave." Ahmed and colleagues also refer to the work of surgeon general of the United States Vivek Murthy, who describes the impact of loneliness on our health in his book *Together*, saying, "Quite simply, human relationship is as essential to our well-being as food and water. Just as hunger and thirst are our body's ways of telling us we need to eat and drink, loneliness is the natural signal that reminds us that we need to connect with other people." Loneliness is every bit as much a bodily experience as it is an emotional one.

We can observe shifts in our own physical and emotional states across social situations in which we do, and conversely, do not feel connected to other people. We may feel physical tension while talking with a difficult colleague or on guard among strangers. But if we are lucky, when we are with our friends and loved ones, we feel bodily tension dissipate. This process of self-regulation happens constantly, within and outside our awareness. Self-regulation is, in part, a matter of physiology—a matter of maintaining bodily functioning. But it is also a response to our sense of safety, of well-being, and of meaning in relation to the people in our lives. It is a constant, iterative process.

In a study conducted in the aftermath of a major hurricane, researchers found that for people living in the affected area, a sense of belonging during the hurricane was a kind of safeguard when it came to symptoms of depression and anxiety after the hurricane. Among people who had withstood the hurricane, they looked at the relationship between perseverative thinking as well as distress *in*tolerance with anxiety and depression and found that those with a stronger sense of belonging fared better than those with a weaker sense of belonging. They argue that a strong sense of belonging is, in fact, a "buffer" and that "high levels of belonging weakened the strong relationship between cognitive vulnerabilities and both depression and anxiety." When we feel that we belong, when we feel, in essence, together with other people, we are less vulnerable to experiences like depression and anxiety.

We learn to self-regulate, but also we are constantly trying to co-regulate. I think, again, of polyvagal theory, at the heart of which is this principle that it is in togetherness that we find safety. And I wonder how it is that co-regulation, that essential human need, aligns with reassurance seeking in the context of anxiety. When we seek out reassurance from other people, we are trying to find a sense of safety. Is this an attempt at co-regulation? Are co-regulation and reassurance seeking two sides of the same coin, or, perhaps, a matter of degree? When I share a particularly absurd worry with my husband, we call it TFN: totally fucking nuts. My anxiety is spoken aloud, aired out, briefly acknowledged, named, but not dwelled upon. It interrupts the cycle, and sometimes it makes me laugh. My thoughts feel less powerful and less toxic—put in their place, just thoughts, after all. I have always been acutely aware of risk and danger—which is to say, terrified of having my heart broken by the agonies the world can inflict upon us—and sometimes just bringing the source of my worry out into the light dispels its power. I'm not alone with it. Still, it's clear to me that what I'm seeking is, largely, reassurance. In our home, this typically takes the form of "You don't think I'm dying, right?" or "Would you have done what I just did?" Perhaps in an ideal world, I would always be able to dispel these worries on my own, without looking to someone else to help me find my way out. Yet this can be incredibly difficult in practice, and sometimes it feels counter to our most human impulses. We are, at our cores, social beings. We want to exist together. We want to share ourselves, and we want to be seen. Surely independence and solitary thinking have their place—but also, we are one another's anchors. Put another way, when I ask, "Would you have done what I just did?" in terms of polyvagal theory, I am also seeking co-regulation. When I ask Porges how the principle of co-regulation in polyvagal theory might inform thinking about reassurance seeking in the context of anxiety, he points out that in the process of co-regulation, we ask, in essence, "Can I trust you enough to give up my defenses?" This is a question we ask one another all our lives.

I recall a patient I treated who wanted desperately to be certain that the pain medication she was prescribed for debilitating back pain in pregnancy had not caused harm to her one-year-old child. But despite reassurance from a series of doctors that this medication was safe, her doubt and fear overwhelmed her. She was terrified that it would be precisely what she had done to care for her own body that would cause irreparable damage to her child's. She spent hours each day reading scientific papers on medication side effects and struggled to enjoy time with her baby or even to sleep. Despite consulting with experts and despite her own research, there was always just enough room for doubt to creep in. Anxiety can create conditions in which no amount of reassurance feels like enough. But maybe we miss something when we see self-regulation, a process that, ideally, takes place alone, within oneself, as the highest goal.

Learning to contain and tolerate distress within oneself is something to aspire to, something to practice. When we rush to quell anxiety by seeking out reassurance from another person, we miss out on the chance to see that we will live through the not-knowing or the uncertainty on our own and that it will not destroy us. Like so many things, reassurance—arguably the most consistently sought remedy for anxiety—isn't all or nothing; rather, it's a matter of degree. Even at the best of times, we look to others to calibrate our experiences and perceptions: we are social creatures, after all, and we are not built to function entirely alone. To seek help from experts, to consult with colleagues, to wonder whether your friend perceives an interaction the way you do—it is healthy, humble, empathic, essential even, to take an interest in how the people around us view things. It is an acknowledgment that your own stance isn't correct simply because it's yours, that the ways in which other people see things matter and can be instructive. But also—at its core, it is human.

We are, in some sense, always holding on to one another. We are social creatures—we exist within families, in friendships, and in other kinds of communities, and we don't function well on our own. Certainly, we can, we should, take responsibility for behaviors and decisions—yet also, we are deeply interdependent. One of our greatest challenges is to see both sides at once. The most profound beauty in our lives exists only in our communion with one another.

Just as anxiety influences the ways we experience love, it has its role when love is lost too. In *Heart: A History*, Sandeep Jauhar, a writer and a cardiologist, says: "There is a heart disorder first recognized about two decades ago called takotsubo cardiomyopathy, or the broken-heart syndrome, in which the heart acutely weakens in response to extreme stress or grief. . . . On an echocardiogram, the heart muscle appears stunned. . . . Takotsubo cardiomyopathy is the archetype of a disease that is controlled by interactions between the emotions and the physical body."

Research consistently links takotsubo cardiomyopathy with anxiety disorders. Among people who are diagnosed with takotsubo cardiomyopathy, there are often prior diagnoses of anxiety disorders. Takotsubo cardiomyopathy is known to happen in the context of grief, following events like the death of a loved one. Grief is not a solely cerebral experience—it reaches into every corner of our being, and it puts massive stress on the entirety of the body, with serious consequences for the heart. We see, in this profoundly literal example, the ways in which, even with so many scientific advances, the heart remains a place where metaphor holds up.

The ties between love and the heart only become stronger. Research supports our intuitive awareness that love, in many forms, is essential and even protective from the start. And we see, too, how it can protect us from some forms of anxiety, or at least take the edge off. New research is beginning to reveal yet another way in which love, in chemical form, protects us. Oxytocin, a naturally occurring hormone in all of our bodies, is known to encourage bonding and feelings of love, and to reduce anxiety. And now it is also being shown to play a part in cardiac healing and regeneration in epicardial cells (which are essential to the functioning of the heart) made from human stem cells, and in zebra fish. In a recently published paper, researchers explained that "our results establish a previously uncharacterized link between OXT (oxytocin) release after cardiac injury and heart regeneration." That is, when the heart is damaged, the body seems to release oxytocin, helping the heart to heal. Will these findings extend fully to humans? It remains to be seen. I'm constantly struggling to shake off my skepticism—and we should maintain a good dose of it—but still, when I read this research, my heart skipped a beat.

⟨⟩

Much is said about the causes of anxiety—whether they are, for instance, biological or social. When we think about anxiety in this way, it is all too easy to fall into a trap of seeing treatment as a process that should correspond directly to one of these sources. If anxiety is biological, then treatment should be medication. If anxiety is social, so too, might treatment be—perhaps therapy, even group therapy. But to take a term from psychoanalysis, anxiety is often overdetermined, meaning that it has many causes. We find the roots of anxiety in the interior workings of our bodies and in our environments, and most of all, in the interactions between the two. Though the intertwining of anxiety and the heart is, medically speaking, well understood, it continues to stretch the boundaries of science, and so our thinking must too.

It's naive, if not patronizing, to call anxiety a gift. But anxiety is revealing, and there is power in it. The heart, in its constant dialogue with the rest of the body and the environment, alerts us to threats ahead and to the less urgent yet nonetheless important anxieties, the kind that stay with us and for which we don't have clear answers. In the face of the uncertainties that anxiety reveals, we look for form and beauty to anchor us to ourselves and to the lives that came before us and the lives that will come after us. When anxiety insists that you get up, how do you stay in your proverbial seat? Stories, love, human connection—these are our anchors.

We know now that the heart doesn't think in the ways it was once believed to. Yet it does, in its way, shape our lives. Across time, our hearts seem to remind us of ourselves in all of our multidimensionality. Despite so many advances in science and medicine, the heart insists that we remember our corporeal nature—the limits and the potential within our bodies—sometimes quietly and sometimes with urgency. And still, the heart remains the symbol it has always been. It stands for feeling and for love. At once a muscle pumping blood throughout the body and a symbol of the most precious parts of life, it reminds us that we are capable of returning to ourselves—and of the connection and the solace that we can have with others. When I feel anxiety creeping in, I remember a period in which my son used to love imaginative play using a children's doctor kit. In our game, which is to say, in the story he was constructing, he would hold his miniature stethoscope to my chest and listen closely, quietly, with gravity. Then I would ask him how my heart sounded. We would lock eyes, protected in our togetherness, and he would look up at me and say, every time, "Still beating!"

Part IV

GUT

7.

INTERCONNECTEDNESS

Sickness is not just an isolated event, or
an unfortunate brush with nature. It is a
form of communication—the language of
the organs—through which nature, society,
and culture speak simultaneously.

—Nancy Scheper-Hughes and Margaret M. Lock,
"The Mindful Body: A Prolegomenon to Future
Work in Medical Anthropology"

Our moods manifest far beyond the confines of our minds. For much of recorded history, the gut has referred to our bodies and to our character. At once a technical term that encompasses the organs that make up the digestive tract, the gut is, too, a symbol of courage. On the surface, the relationship between anxiety and the gut is obvious and well accepted. It is a commonly held belief that anxiety brings about or otherwise exacerbates gut problems. Moments of worry or panic tend to reveal themselves in our guts—whether as butterflies in the stomach or changes in appetite, or, in some cases, as chronic gastrointestinal illness. And in fact, these are very old ideas. We can look to Chinese medicine, in which acupuncture, whose history dates back thousands of years, addressed the relationship between gut health and other aspects of our well-being, or to Ayurvedic medicine's attention to gut health. More recently, medical historian Ian Miller has written about the ways that people over the course of history have known that our guts and our feelings are linked. He points to the work of, for instance, Robert Whytt, an eighteenth-century physician from Scotland, who "developed the concept of 'nervous sympathy' to describe the mechanisms which he believed connected the inner body organs" and also writes that in Victorian medicine, "the stomach appeared . . . to occupy a central and persistent position in the development of key fields of medicine including pathological anatomy, physiology, surgery and psychosomatic medicine." So we see that people have long understood that our guts and our minds are in constant conversation. Now, research on the functioning of the gut is beginning to shed light on the precise nature of the communication that goes on between our guts and our brains, and we see that things aren't so straightforward. It turns out that the gut is part of our emotional functioning, not simply reactive to it.

We live amid worlds of influence that are invisible to the naked eye but that have massive sway over our lives. Research on the gut tends to evoke science fiction more than it does science. It is a world of its own that we are coming to see with new clarity, a wonderous world inside of us. I imagine how it may have felt when, in the sixteenth century, the microscope emerged, or three centuries later, with the beginnings of germ theory, or even in the early days of quantum mechanics—suddenly, there is so much more. A world, previously unseen, alive.

ℰ

When my son was about five months old, I got a call at work from his daycare, that there had been a bottle mix-up. He had accidentally been fed another woman's breastmilk. The daycare was horrified. I was horrified. And though I knew, as a matter of basic logic, that this was not reversible, I called his pediatrician, who told me, essentially, that nothing needed to be done. (And I say to myself now, what exactly did I think one could do anyway?) Still horrified, I told a dear friend at work, also a mother to small children. She said I should be thrilled—"Think of his microbiome! You should ask them to do it every week!" And I laughed. I laugh thinking about it now. I laugh not only because of the absurdity of it all—at the thought that something could have been done, at my friend's reaction. But now I think, too, about the ways that this mix-up reflects larger, deeply fixed ideas of control and contamination when it comes to the body, and when it comes to the worlds that we construct within our bodies. In fact, in scientific writing about the microbiome a social language emerges. Terms like "community richness" and "microbial communities." Amazing! They describe the state of our microbiome and, too, they reflect states that we aspire to—states in which we commune with others. The vocabulary of the microbiome points toward the unseen life within our bodies. And it provokes questions too: How independent are our bodies from those closest to us? To what extent are we separate from the environments in which we live? It turns out, not very.

Since the start of the COVID-19 pandemic, we've come to experience other people, other places, as dirty, viral, literally coated in risk, threatening in a way that, for many, they hadn't previously been. Certainly, this sense of other people as a source of potential contamination has been especially vexing for people with anxiety. Anxiety disorders, and OCD in particular, often include fears of contamination, of dirtiness. For those who regularly fight themselves on this point, at the start of the pandemic there was a sudden, massive, literally worldwide reinforcement of their fears. Buttons were pushed, if you will. We came to see safety through a lens of separation. Our interconnectedness—from the ways that we provide essential services like physical care and education to our deeply social nature as a species, quite simply, our need to be with one another, fell under new scrutiny, and felt, were, for a time, a real liability, a threat. We came to crave the warmth of human contact. And even as March 2020 recedes further into the past, we are changed, I suspect, forever. Looking back, our interconnectedness takes on new dimensions of meaning, from the ways in which we understand our bodily well-being to the ways that we nurture ourselves and one another.

ら

We know now that the gut's response to anxiety and fear is utilitarian in that it is one of the ways that the body prepares for fight or flight (that, for instance, the bowels can slow or empty in a state of emergency). We know, too, that the evolutionary value of this gut response to anxiety no longer aligns with most of our modern circumstances. So it is that we've come, over generations, to attempt to ignore our guts. We learn to brush off a nervous stomach or an internal sense that something isn't right. We avoid the questions the gut asks. We struggle with our guts.

The gut encompasses the parts of our bodies that most often elicit disgust and shame—the digestive system, from top to tail. Children understand from an early age that there is something taboo about the functioning of the gut—that it is for private spaces only. They often use so-called bathroom humor—and in this way, they test the limits of the taboo. We use terms like "spilling one's guts" to describe an outpouring of information, and the words imply a potentially regrettable loss of control.

For as much as we try to look away from our guts, we've actually been subject to, and benefited from, research on fecal matter during the COVID-19 pandemic too. Scientists have consistently found that they can look to wastewater for information about where COVID outbreaks are taking place. The contents of our guts hold a great deal of information about the future of our health as individuals and as communities—information that we have either discounted or chosen to ignore, relegated to taboo.

Over the past few decades, the gut has come to be referred to as the "second brain," a term introduced by neurobiologist Michael Gershon. Gershon writes: "We should care about our second brain for the same reasons we care about our first. Descartes may have said 'I think therefore I am,' but he only said that because his guts let him. The brain in the bowel has got to work right or no one will have the luxury to think at all." We know now that the gut is implicated in many of the functions of the body that were previously associated solely with the brain—most of all, our emotional lives. And perhaps more remarkably, the brain and gut don't function in isolation—rather, they work in tandem, alongside the microbiome, via the microbiota-gut-brain axis, and in this way, their workings have massive impact on our physical and emotional health. Gershon and colleague Kara Gross Margolis evoke that social language of the gut when they explain: "The interaction between the microbiota, the bowel, and the brain . . . is an ongoing, tripartite conversation." Cutting-edge research on our "second brain" is exciting and hugely promising because it is taking on the multidirectional nature of the ways in which our microbiomes, our guts, and our brains interact.

It turns out that not only do the brain and gut communicate with and influence each other, they contain some of the same essential parts—neurotransmitters. Neurotransmitters are molecules that we often hear about in the context of mental health treatment—substances like serotonin and dopamine. The term "neurotransmitter" refers to the nervous system (the brain, the spinal cord, the nerves), but actually, neurotransmitters are also produced in the gut. The vast majority of the serotonin in our bodies and some 50 percent of our dopamine, both of which are central to our mood, are produced in the enteric nervous system, which is that "second brain" that the gut is often described as.

The microbiome refers to "the community of microorganisms . . . that exists in a particular environment." The gut microbiome is now the subject of a great deal of research and has emerged into the mainstream—both in medicine and in popular culture. It's become clear, indeed backed by data, that the microbiome has massive implications for our health—for gastrointestinal conditions, yes, but also for conditions like rheumatoid arthritis, Alzheimer's disease, and even anxiety disorders.

From birth to death, interactions between our bodies and the world shape and reshape our microbiomes. During birth, as a baby passes through the vaginal canal, they pick up the bacteria that forms their mother's microbiome. In *I Contain Multitudes: The Microbes Within Us and a Grander View of Life,* Ed Yong writes, "When each baby is born, it leaves the sterile world of its mother's womb and is immediately colonized by her vaginal microbes; almost three-quarters of a newborn's strains can be traced directly back to its mother." So we see that the layers of biological inheritance that form us are made up of far more than our genes. In this initial passage, it is the physical contact between baby and mother, between one body and another, a primal interconnectedness, that begins to shape the gut.

But of course, not all babies are born via the vaginal canal, and while cesarean sections are an essential, life-saving procedure in many instances, they are also associated with higher rates of obesity, asthma, and respiratory-tract infections in children—and some researchers think this could be due to differences in the microbiome. Because the initial passage through the vaginal canal seems to be a pivotal step in the development of the microbiome, doctors and scientists are developing workarounds to replace it. Vaginal seeding is a procedure that can be used during births via C-section in which a mother's vaginal fluids are transferred, on sterile gauze, onto the skin of their baby. It sounds too good to be true—that such a simple solution could have any real impact. But research suggests that it could be an effective means of helping along a baby's developing microbiome. Indeed, a recent study found that when comparing babies born via C-section who did and didn't undergo vaginal seeding, those who did developed microbiomes that bore greater resemblance to babies born via vaginal birth.

So much seems to happen at the start, long before we have any concept of our microbiomes or any control over the factors that shape them. Recent research suggests that, as with so many aspects of human development, those earliest years of life, particularly until around age three, matter quite a lot for the formation of the microbiome, and, in turn, may hold sway over our long-term health. It's not that we aren't capable of degrees of change later in life (or after age three!) but rather that the structures that develop in our first years can become far more difficult to shift later on. As a psychologist and as a parent, this idea that we, as humans, are subject to periods in which certain kinds of learning and development are possible, but that these periods are limited—this is a hard pill to swallow. The term "critical period" refers to a window of time in which certain kinds of development are possible—like, for instance, some aspects of language learning—and this is a window that, at some point, closes for good. "Sensitive periods" are times in which certain kinds of development are optimal, yet they could still occur later. Whether or not you think in terms of critical and sensitive periods, this concept lives within us all. As we reflect on our own lives, as we reflect on what happened, or what didn't happen, we face the limits of our own plasticity. Our guts, too, are subject to these possibilities and to these limits.

Research on adults suggests that the gut microbiome may be fundamentally different in people with symptoms of anxiety relative to those without symptoms of anxiety. Recent studies have found that people with symptoms of anxiety have, for instance, less gut microbiome diversity than those without symptoms of anxiety. One of these research teams also found, in a small sample of people with GAD, that even when anxiety symptoms improved, the gut microbiome remained imbalanced. But research in this area is far from conclusive. A systematic review of studies on the relationship between the gut microbiome and symptoms of anxiety and depression found that results in this field are inconsistent and don't point in one clear direction. However, they did find that both anxiety and depression were associated with "a higher relative abundance of proinflammatory species," meaning more of the gut bacteria that may promote inflammation in the body rather than reduce it.

When I read research on the microbiome and mental health, despite its currently inconclusive status, I feel a need come over me to change my lifestyle, my diet—urgently. To eat more fermented foods. To eliminate sugar. If I'm careful enough, always thinking of my insides, putting pleasure aside, maybe I will evade dementia, or rheumatoid arthritis, or cancer. But usually, when this happens, it feels less like science and more like fear. That here is a catastrophe I could, with enough vigilance, prevent. When I slow things down, when that fearful edge wears off, reality shows itself. Catastrophes don't work this way.

Our guts seem to overflow with meaning, even in the ways we speak about them. But somehow, I find it difficult to keep my gut in my mind. We are often quick to skip over the emotional underpinnings of the gut. I remind myself, with some effort, that this is, in fact, how the body works. That this isn't hocus-pocus—it is science. I know that I am not alone in this. Despite so much research on the links between the gut and the mind, there remains an air of skepticism, even in clinical circles. Questions circle around whether or not it is possible, at this point, to use knowledge of the gut-brain connection practically, around what can be done with these (albeit exciting) new findings. I attended a lecture a few years ago in which a psychiatrist described prescribing probiotics alongside psychiatric medications for some of her patients with anxiety and depression. I remember feeling deeply skeptical, and I detected a similar response in the faces of my colleagues. My skepticism was not about the relationship between the brain and the gut—I have no doubts about the powerful ties that link our guts and our brains. Rather, I struggle with the question of whether we are able to influence these ties, given the limits of current science. To what degree do we have any real power over our guts? Are we or will we soon be capable of harnessing the workings of the gut in the interest of psychological well-being? Will treating the gut, addressing the state of the microbiome, cross the threshold from the worlds of research and health-food stores into standard practice? What happens when we change our diets to improve gut health? Or when we take probiotics? Will these changes amount to something, which is to say, will they change our bodies and, in so doing, our health, our lives? Or is it like spitting in the wind?

These are open questions, and they evoke strong responses, with believers on both sides. I want to know: How plastic is the gut? How much change are we really capable of—and what kinds of changes are worth making? We know that our bodies can undergo some kinds of change—we can, say, build muscle—but not all kinds of change; our forms are dictated in part by our genetics. Change is possible, but there are limits. But then, what is changeable is plastic in its own way. Changes that were previously thought impossible are now part of ordinary life.

We think of the things we put into our bodies, things like food, as within our control, to some degree. But so much of what seems to shape mental health, and the gut especially, comes from the environments in which we exist, with innumerable factors outside our individual control. A recent study looked at how difficult experiences early in life (like abuse in childhood) may impact mental health later on. Researchers found that "ELA (early life adversity) can lead to persistent disruptions in the brain-gut system, which may contribute to susceptibility to psychological conditions later into adulthood"—conditions like depression and anxiety. Over and over, psychological research points back. So much seems to depend on the earliest days and years of our lives. We see the importance of the environments to which we are exposed. Of early attachment to caregivers. The luck we are born into, or not. These are linked factors—they are an interconnectedness that we do not choose—and, alongside our genetics, they manifest in our bodies, sometimes right away and sometimes many years down the road. Even in instances in which children are well cared for, even in the best of times, nothing, nobody is perfect. So much weight is placed on those first years, when, in childhood, our lives are at the whim of our caretakers, or as parents, we feel wildly novice. The importance of our beginnings, backed by research and finding its way toward popular culture, helps us to see that we are indeed shaped from the start.

It can feel as though our first years are a prophecy—but they aren't. In anxious times, what begins as an appreciation for the development that takes place in our first years—in our brains, our guts—can morph into perfectionism and obsessional worry. We can imagine that maybe, with enough effort, we can control the formation of our children. That if we do all things just so, if we're on all the time, our child will grow up in perfect health, with a microbiome to beat all microbiomes, invulnerable to disease, invulnerable to anxiety, invulnerable to life itself. Each day, when my son comes home from school, he eats a piece of candy, or as he puts it, "a sweetie." This is not in line with the microbiome-centered diet that some research supports. But he looks forward to it, and it eases the transition from school to home, so if I'm honest, I lean on it. And even more so, restriction and rigidity have costs too.

Troubles with anxiety and one's gut are often attributed to a failure of strength and seen as a sign of internal flimsiness. If anxiety shows itself in your gastrointestinal system, if, say, your anxiety is accompanied by a stomachache or nausea or diarrhea, you might be said to have a *weak* stomach. This line of thinking implies (at least) two things: that anxiety exercises influence over the stomach, and that anxiety is a flaw in one's character, one that results in a kind of frailty. But research suggests that this sort of explanation comes up short—that, in fact, anxiety and the gut operate on a two-way street. There is a growing body of evidence that suggests that the mutual influence between the brain and the gut may manifest in the form of anxiety and certain medical conditions. A recent meta-analysis looked at the relationship between symptoms of anxiety and depression and inflammatory bowel disease, which brings with it symptoms like abdominal pain and weight loss and sometimes requires surgery and hospitalization. They found "significant bi-directional effects of brain-gut interactions in patients with IBD," meaning that anxiety and depression were linked to later worsening of inflammatory bowel disease, but also inflammatory bowel disease was linked to symptoms of anxiety and depression later on. Our emotional and physical well-being are in intimate dialogue with each other.

The relationship between anxiety and the gut is etched deeply within us. A massive genetic study looking at the link between irritable bowel syndrome (IBS) and anxiety disorders found clear *genetic* associations between anxiety and IBS. There are "shared pathogenic pathways, rather than, for example, anxiety causing abdominal symptoms." This research points instead toward a shared origin story for anxiety and IBS. And though this study focused on IBS, it begets larger, as-of-yet unanswerable questions: Where does anxiety begin? In the body, or in the world?

Now that we have evidence of these differences in the gut, and data to hold us up (rather than relying on anecdotal observations of links between gastrointestinal symptoms and anxiety), what can be done? This is where the rubber tends to meet the road. In many ways, our understanding seems to exceed our tools. Although this is almost always true in science and medicine, it can be heartbreaking. We know, for instance, that plaques appear in the brains of people with Alzheimer's disease, yet treatment remains in a nascent stage. We know, too, that a proliferation of abnormal cells gives rise to cancer—yet treatment remains imperfect and sometimes painfully crude. This same logic applies when it comes to mental health. Our knowledge of bodily systems is years ahead of our ability to change them.

In a wild, almost unbelievable twist: fecal transplants. Fecal transplants are what they sound like. Research on fecal transplants looks at the effects of literally transplanting fecal matter from one person's body, that is presumed to be healthy, to another, who is in need of treatment, so far mainly for gastrointestinal problems. The transplant can come in the form of a capsule that is swallowed or it can be placed via enema or colonoscopy. In fact, they aren't a new idea. Fecal transplants, in slightly different forms, are thought to have existed as far back as fourth-century China. Fecal transplants struck me as utterly absurd just a few years ago. But also, just as they bump up against taboo, they remind us that we, our bodies, our well-being, are powerfully interconnected. That it is through the worlds that exist within us that we have the potential to restore one another. Will it one day be commonplace to take capsules of fecal matter to treat anxiety? It is hard for me to imagine—but then, I also thought that texting would never last; it struck me as absurd, inefficient, and totally impractical.

Obviously grotesque, we stay away from fecal matter—and certainly we don't eat shit. The thought alone evokes a primal sense of disgust, one that is, in the most basic sense, a survival mechanism. But fecal transplants have been shown to be strikingly helpful in treating some illnesses—like Clostridium difficile infection, a bacterial infection that affects the colon and can cause serious, at times life-threatening, illness. Research suggests that fecal transplants are also useful for treating ulcerative colitis (UC). UC is an inflammatory bowel disease that is chronic and painful. It includes symptoms like abdominal cramping, bleeding, diarrhea, and nausea. Like IBS, it is often associated with anxiety and other mood symptoms. Given the close ties between the brain and the gut, scientists are beginning to look at the effects of fecal transplants on mental health. Research, though in its very early stages, is beginning to find evidence of improvement of depression following fecal transplants. When it comes to anxiety, a review of research on fecal transplants for psychiatric illness found that anxiety symptoms also seem to improve following fecal transplants. What's more, this review also looked at research on fecal transplants in mice, which found that fecal transplants may work both ways: mice exhibiting anxious and depressive behaviors seemed to improve following fecal transplants from nonanxious mice, and anxious and depressive behaviors seemed to be transmitted when fecal transplants were given from anxious mice to nonanxious mice. These findings are impressive, exciting—like finding a key to a door that's been locked for a very long time. Soon after, members of the same research team conducted a small study in which they looked at the effects of "microbial ecosystem therapy"—a treatment taken in capsule form that was made of "40 strains of bacteria that were purified and lab-grown from the stool of a single healthy donor." The treatment was associated with an improvement in symptoms of depression and anxiety, at which point I feel myself reaching for my phone to text my beloved group chat of therapist friends. But then, my own skeptical tendencies aside, we must remember: these are early days and very small studies. There's a long way between a mouse and a human. And in studies with human subjects, improvements in depression and anxiety often seemed to wear off in the months following the transplant.

I spoke to my friend Travis Gibson, PhD, an assistant professor at Harvard Medical School and a principal investigator at Brigham and Women's Hospital who studies host-microbiome interactions, about how to think about fecal transplants today. We talked about the long history of fecal transplants—from the "yellow soup" described in fourth-century China, to more modern iterations. Gibson explained to me that to use fecal transplants today, scientists look for a "defined community" of microbes—something knowable and specific—a substance that has the potential to function like a drug. And I imagine a social event, a wedding, maybe, one in which disparate communities, some "defined," intermingle and then merge. I asked Gibson, too, about where he stands on probiotics. I tell him about my reading in the field and my own ambivalence, manifest in my own inconsistency in taking them. He says "we need delivery mechanisms where the probiotics could actually work, where you could deliver something *alive*"—because probiotics often don't survive the journey to our guts. I ask him if he takes probiotics, and he says he doesn't. But then, he tells me that he gives them to his son when he is sick. In myself and in our conversation, in the research in front of me, I hear it: *maybe, it's possible, someday, just in case.*

We come next to the things that we put into our guts—what we eat and drink (or don't), from food to supplements. Nutrition occupies a troublesome place when it comes to health, mental and otherwise. On one hand, the idea, the fact, that the food we eat matters for our well-being seems obvious, barely worth stating. It is something we can feel. Yet on the other, we (myself ever so much included) tend to treat nutrition with skepticism and to minimize its role when it comes to the ways we see our health. To change one's relationship with food requires a gradual and constant effort. But most of all, food stands for so much more than nourishment. To change what and how we eat is to push up against routine, comfort, history, privilege, economics, even desire itself.

Effects of nutrition on health, mental and otherwise, are notoriously difficult to study. Our diets are not easily isolated from other aspects of our lives, and the things that we eat are not so easily managed as, say, a single medication in a research setting. Yet we know that food matters enormously for our well-being and that differences in the foods we eat can change the course of our health altogether. In a recent look at the data, researchers reviewed studies on the impact of diet on mental health, including anxiety disorders. They noted the inconclusive nature of many studies but also put forth recommendations taking into consideration the larger picture on anxiety and nutrition. In particular, they point to the importance of a healthy diet (one that includes fruits and vegetables, fatty fish, and vitamins like zinc, magnesium, and vitamin C) in addressing anxiety disorders. Some scientists even view anxiety disorders as a form of metabolic disease, and they see anxiety as having to do with inflammation and problems with the gut. A recent paper from this vantage point presented nutritional recommendations as a component of treatment for anxiety. They argue that to improve microbiome health and reduce inflammation in the body, it is best to remove gluten and artificial sweeteners from one's diet and to be sure to consume omega-3s, turmeric, and vitamin D, while also following a ketogenic diet (a diet that is low in carbohydrates and high in protein and fat). To argue that dietary changes could be a way to relieve anxiety—this is bold. And it's attractive. Nutritional recommendations can provide a (usually temporary) sense of control and agency over symptoms that feel entirely undermining and out of control. Could I, could the anxious among us, exorcise our anxieties through these sorts of dietary changes? Could everything I need be in the grocery store?

I'm skeptical. In part, my skepticism comes from a rational place. But also, in my heart of hearts, I fear that even if I, if one, were to follow these dietary recommendations to the letter, it might not be enough. That changes like these might not be sufficiently potent to stand up to the worst that anxiety has to offer. And more importantly, I worry that we might be missing the point. When we think of anxiety as a metabolic disease, it feels so deeply, so entirely physical, so akin to a condition like diabetes. And although I see value and at least partial truth in this approach, I find that through an entirely biological lens, it becomes a bit too easy to see anxiety as a straight line, with its origins solely, instead of partially, in the body.

Along with dietary recommendations, we're now seeing supplements—probiotics in particular—being promoted as a means to reduce symptoms of anxiety. Researchers tend to think of probiotics as a possible *component* of treatment for mental illness rather than a stand-alone approach—and this nuance often gets lost in public conversation. We're not talking about probiotics as a panacea for anxiety, or at least we shouldn't be. The term "psychobiotics" refers to the use of probiotics to treat symptoms of mental illness, and it's become an area of massive interest as we understand more about the interactions of the brain and the gut. But there are layers of questions at play. Do psychobiotics change the gut itself? And then, if they do, are they powerful enough to bring about tangible changes in anxiety symptoms, changes that impact people's daily lives? Evidence is mixed at best as to whether or not probiotics may be able to reduce anxiety. A recent meta-analysis found no meaningful changes in anxiety following probiotic use. And in another review of research on probiotic use in the context of mental illness, researchers found that there just isn't enough solid research currently available on the effects of probiotics on anxiety, and that which does exist is quite limited.

This is a conversation that forces us to think about what is now, and what could one day be. If you ask me, today, in 2024, if probiotics treat anxiety, I will tell you that as of now, the evidence suggests that they do not—at least not enough to make a real dent in it. Not enough to change your life. But even so, when I read research on psychobiotics, I feel hopeful (as I make a note to buy some while eating a peanut butter cup). We're limited by our current technologies, by our current understandings, but also I believe we're onto something powerful.

One of the more problematic aspects of psychology as a field is the tendency to see approaches to treatment in all-or-nothing terms (ironic considering most forms of therapy aim, in some way, to reduce this kind of thinking). So often, clinicians argue that their own preferred method of treatment (cognitive-behavioral therapy, say, or psychodynamic psychotherapy) is the only way forward. There can be a sense of diametric opposition, a digging in of heels. That scientists aren't, as of yet, shouting from the rooftops about the power of dietary changes to reduce anxiety does not mean that nutrition doesn't matter. And though we can't rely solely on nutrition or supplements to treat anxiety, we can continue to see them as part of the picture, as worth our investigation. It seems to me that all signs point in a similar, reasonable direction: Generally speaking, eating well, and eating with some understanding of our gut health, is good for us, even if we can't change the course of our lives entirely through doing so.

It's important to remember that many things are worth doing even when research has yet to explain them. When we think about the impact of the things that we, quite literally, incorporate, we tend to think first of food and supplements. But so much of what finds its way into our bodies is less tangible than a vegetable or a candy bar. Things like fear or comfort or even love—they, too, exert influence, and have physical, even measurable, implications for our bodies. There is wisdom in seeing subtlety and wisdom in recognizing the limits of our control, down to the ways that the things that we eat, and our experiences, work within our bodies.

When my father was diagnosed with early-onset Alzheimer's disease, I, like so many of us do, went immediately into a state of wondering what might be done—a more tolerable frame of mind than the fear and despair that were clawing at me. We learned about his diagnosis as I was writing this chapter, so I'd been thinking about how nutrition impacts the gut and the brain for some time. Reading in this field, I came across study after study pointing to the ways in which a Mediterranean diet supports brain health, and noting that it is recommended for people with conditions including Alzheimer's disease, without realizing how personally relevant these papers would soon come to feel.

As soon as my father's diagnosis was confirmed, I sent him a slew of Mediterranean-diet cookbooks. As I placed the order, it felt truly urgent, like overnight shipping wasn't fast enough. I then called my sister and told her, bossily, terrified, that we would need to be on this diet too. We would need to think ahead. When my husband got home that evening, I told him that we would now be following a strict Mediterranean diet—meaning starting this instant. He (kindly, gently) pointed out that most of the time, we already do. But in my desperation to solve, desperation to prevent (one that I've yet to entirely let go of), "most of the time" struck me as sickeningly inadequate. The next day, my mom told me that when she heard the news, she'd sent my dad and stepmom a panettone (a sweet Italian bread), and she felt terrible that it could pose a temptation, a violation of recommendations to stay away from sugar, as though the panettone would make the difference. I've said it before and I'll say it again—I didn't lick it off the street.

But then, none of us is so consistent, so pure, so perfect in our ways. Soon after my dietary declaration, it was Christmas. I ate all sorts of things that fell outside my plan—we all did. I told myself that what matters most is what we do most of the time. That the holidays are special, they are to be enjoyed. That this holiday had a particular poignancy to it for my family.

But lingering below remains this question: Could I be good enough, stay in line enough, to prevent all disasters, to change the course of a diagnosis? Could I endow my father with health, could I rid his brain, his gut of inflammation? Could I rid us all of fear and dread? No. I know that I cannot. I know that it is anxiety that pushes me into this place, rather than reason. That what we do most of the time *is* what counts, that there is no point in striving for perfection—

no gains, really, to be had, and certainly no joy. What can we change, but more so, what must we accept? That we are human, that life gets in the way, that, in fact, we can only hope that life will get in the way. After all, a life that revolves entirely around maintaining perfect routines, that is a very sad life indeed. That here, as with all things, we can't have complete control, and much remains uncertain. That, whatever you believe, whatever you take on—whether, in the service of reducing anxiety, or of changing your gut or your mind, we are doing our best.

Research on the gut evokes an ecological mood. I think of vaginal seeding. Of community richness. With a glimpse of our guts, we see that there may be profound value in cultivating them—whether through diet or supplements or even, maybe one day, fecal matter. We want desperately to cultivate our insides—to be stronger, more resilient. But as much as we strive to alter our biology—to bring about that diversity in our gut microbiomes that seems to portend health in the gut and the brain—we also crave changes in the ways we experience ourselves in the world. In the ways we interact and relate to other people, and most of all, to ourselves. So, what does it really mean to be someone who has guts? When it comes down to it, our guts depend upon, and flourish within, our interconnectedness, our shared experience. When anxiety shines a light on risk, when it screams the potential for contagion, for contamination, it isolates, it turns us inward. Our guts remind us that things are not so simple— that we are of the world, and that we cannot live in isolation. Sometimes, when we are lucky, good things are contagious too. There is little opportunity for cultivation without risking a bit of contagion, a bit of contamination. We are all profoundly connected, down to the sewage that flows below our feet. To live with guts is to take on this interconnectedness, to see the potential in it. We see that in the transmission of fecal matter, the gut changes, sometimes for the better. What if we were to share another sort of guts with one another? It turns out that we can look inward and outward at once.

Years ago (in a conversation about relationships, not the microbiome), a dear friend pointed out that there is an entire world within another person, and I've thought about it many times since. Within each of us, no matter how it may seem, no matter our limitations, there are worlds, and it is in the interactions among these worlds that life is lived. The gut is this way too. It reminds us that there are dimensions of influence between our bodies, the people in our lives, and our surrounds that we have yet to appreciate. It is in the intermingling of these worlds that we find strength and beauty in one another, and, ideally, that we create a profound sort of safety with one another, one that reminds us that when it comes to those deepest fears, the anxieties that keep us up at night, what we have is each other—that really, there is no other way. That we must be humble and curious. When you feel the edge of another world approaching, that grandest sort of interconnectedness, just before you can make out its contours—this is wonder. A hungriness, a luminosity, a thing to cultivate.

8.

TRUST AND AGENCY

How should a person be?

—Sheila Heti, *How Should a Person Be?*

The gut consists, quite literally, of our insides, but it is also symbolic of those most internal parts of ourselves—of our vulnerability, our courage, our instincts, of what is most true to us. We know that feelings of anxiety manifest powerfully in our guts, and that our bodies suffer the consequences. But most of us also experience times in which anxiety, along with our gut, helps us to see that something is awry. A dangerous situation is avoided, or a much-needed change at work is made. A relationship is seen with new-found clarity. The gut is a way toward a kind of self-understanding that cuts to the core.

For as much as we seem to struggle with our guts, we revere them, after the fact. When we find that our gut protected us, we feel a righteous sort of pride. To follow one's gut, to have the guts, to be gutsy—these are things to aspire to. To act with guts requires us to pay attention to our innermost thoughts, however uncomfortable they make us feel. The gut, perhaps more than any other part of the body, reminds us—sometimes with symptoms we are aware of, like nausea, and sometimes in imperceptible shifts that nonetheless impact our health, say, changes to the microbiome as a consequence of chronic stress—that we cannot escape ourselves.

When we talk about guts, we are talking about risk, responsibility, control, and then, agency. Our relationship to each of these forces gives shape to our days—from the ways we approach our personal lives to our work. They impact our decision-making, and they determine the extent to which we are able to live according to our own values. Anxiety shines a bright light on each of our idiosyncratic ways of relating to these gut senses. Potential risks may overshadow potential benefits. Feelings of responsibility may rise in excess, while power in one's own life may seem to diminish. Where one might look to gut feelings, to those deepest instincts, to move forward, there is, instead, friction and overwhelming uncertainty.

I'm reminded of a patient I treated who came to therapy because she was having panic attacks and had developed insomnia seemingly out of nowhere. But as treatment unfolded, it became clear that her anxiety was years in the making. She felt she'd arrived at middle age having made decisions on the basis of how she felt she *should* live, which was based on the expectations and the wants of others—in her professional trajectory, in her relationship, even in her decision to have children. Her family's needs and her professional obligations seemed to subsume her awareness of her own desires, from how to spend a long weekend to how she would spend her retirement.

When push comes to shove, we have to know our gut. When you

ignore your gut, you miss out on essential information about what it is that matters most to you. It is a slippery slope—in this way, you can become too easily swayed by other people, and over time you may find yourself in situations you are unhappy with, which feel like the product of constant reaction rather than choice. These moments accumulate, and over time life becomes smaller, and bearings are lost. When you understand how it is that you relate to risk, to responsibility, and to agency—that is, when you come to know your gut—you can make decisions in accordance with it. Instead of being driven by anxiety, you can instead act with self-possession. In finding and knowing your gut, you come to feel the ground beneath yourself. You come to see what you want, who you are, and who you want to be. It's a kind of power.

I find that sometimes I'm bold and insistent. I follow my instincts, and I feel the power of having done so, like a force coursing through my body. I feel, quite literally, stronger. But then, sometimes I feel small. I let go of things, of thoughts, of positions that I wish I had held on to. I fail to speak up for myself, or I end an interaction knowing that I have been steamrolled. This is true for many of us—and it tends to vary by circumstance. For some people, it's easier to stay with oneself at work than with family, for instance, while for others, it's the opposite. We want consistency from ourselves, but when it comes to acting according to our guts, we are, for better and for worse, subject to our histories and to present influence. There can be a momentary, false sense of relief when we succumb to anxiety, when we avoid, when we kick the can down the road. But usually it is followed by a sickening sense of having forsaken oneself. In moments when anxiety tempts me to postpone, to say less, or to be smaller, I observe its weight, its place in my decision-making. I try, instead, to turn (stumble) inward, to make decisions with my gut in my mind. In the right light, risk, responsibility, agency—they all feel like guts.

But there are those people who seem to have guts come hell or high water. One of my dearest friends, who is also a psychologist— her guts blow me away, they are one of the many things I love about her. Over the years, I've seen her stand up to formidable adversaries many times, and her guts exceed her anxiety every time. She is un- wavering. When things aren't right, she says so, and this includes when things are not right within herself. She will not allow herself to be diminished.

I call my friend to talk to her about her guts. I tell her that I'm writing about the gut—and about having guts. I tell her that I want to understand how her gut is so powerful, how, psychologically speaking, it works—for my book, and also, let's be honest, I want to learn for my own benefit—which, of course, she knows. She reminds me that her guts are not in lieu of anxiety. She tells me that for her, the anxiety that comes with the thought of leaving unsaid that which needs to be said is in and of itself propulsive. That for her, this anxi- ety is greater than any fear of saying too much, being too bold. This is how I want to be. Because exercising one's guts, anxiety be damned, this is a way to see things—and to see oneself—clearly.

It turns out: anxiety is not the opposite of guts.

ↅ

Early in my clinical training, I was both surprised and relieved to find that when you are trained in psychotherapy (and, too, as a patient in psychotherapy), one's instincts are considered valuable, even informative. Rather than being seen as hocus-pocus or feelings to be ignored in favor of that which is expressed in words alone, they are a kind of data. Despite my incredible fortune to have the family and friends that I have, I, like so many others, had grown up treating my instincts with a heavy dose of skepticism. But in clinical training, we learned to notice and describe our internal reactions to our work with patients. Information that I would previously have discarded as unempirical began to shed light on important dynamics playing out that I hadn't previously articulated. Anxiety became something to notice, and those instinctive feelings that I had yet to fully understand were worthy of attention rather than something to stifle. In this way, I came, little by little, to trust my instincts, and I learned that while there are plenty of feelings that we don't as of yet have data to describe satisfactorily, that doesn't mean that they aren't important.

When you are prone to anxiety, it can become difficult to sort out what is gut instinct and what is anxiety. It becomes useful, crucial even, to determine which is which. Is your urge to leave the party early a gut instinct that you should heed? Is it an awareness that something is awry that has yet to become fully clear to you, yet to be translated into words? Or, is this urge actually a reflection of feeling anxious among new colleagues? The ever-evolving art is in knowing the difference between the two.

As powerful as gut feelings can be, like anxiety, they are not a form of fortune-telling. Research in psychology and political science consistently shows that most of us are not much good at predicting the future—whether we are attempting to predict the success of a business or political events or others' future violent behavior. Nor are we very good at accurately predicting how we will *feel* in the future, a process known as affective forecasting. One might, for instance, anticipate feeling anxious at a party and come to find that they enjoy themselves, or look forward to the Christmas holiday and come to find themselves exhausted and craving routine. And thank goodness. This is the blessing and the curse of anxiety—we can't be sure what will happen in the world around us or in our innermost selves. But also, we don't have to be sure—it's not possible.

There is a well-known idea, one that is wise and worth remembering, that often, the things that most devastate us, that become pivotal points in our lives, are not those that we've worried about for years. Rather, these turning points tend to surprise us, and in this way, they remind us of the absurdity of so many of our worries. We are forced to face this proof that our worry is neither predictive nor preventative. Our anxiety is, most often, an ill-conceived exercise against chaos. It is easy to forget that under the specter of anxiety, most of our worries say more about our internal turmoil than they do about the future.

That said, I find that when I pay close attention, gut instincts feel different from anxiety. They are less frantic and made up more of knowledge than of questions. Rather than fear of what might be, it is as though it is already done.

Years ago, I was riding the subway on the way home from work. A woman seated near me was drinking a bottle of water, and as I sat there, I imagined her throwing the water in my face. A few seconds later, the train stopped short and the water flew out of the open bottle, onto the floor.

A handful of times, in the car with my family, I've had a sense come over me that something is about to go wrong on the road, and I've warned my husband to drive especially carefully, to keep some extra space around us. A minute later, as we sit in traffic, we witness a fender bender a few cars ahead. Or a car changes lanes too quickly. We agree that this is very strange. Plenty of seemingly irrational (or at least inexplicable) feelings seem to protect us.

My husband tells me I've gotten "witchier" since our son was born. I think he's right.

These kinds of experiences are not easily explained, nor quantified, with data. What, exactly, am I picking up on before the water spills on the floor or the car stops short? From a rational standpoint, I tell myself, there are surely signals outside my conscious awareness that are at play, influencing my perception. Maybe in these moments, I'm noticing an acceleration of the cars around us, or brake lights turning on, without putting two and two together. But still, I can't seem to put my finger on it. And as much as these experiences seem to derive from somewhere deep in my gut, they are also accompanied by some anxiety. Sometimes, a sense of knowing can be unsettling. It can feel like too much information, too soon. In this way, anxiety and gut feelings remain, for most of us, intertwined, never entirely distinct.

These gut feelings, so to speak, are fairly common phenomena, and they have been examined and interpreted for thousands of years, across many cultures. But their predictive quality remains slippery and largely unexplainable. In 2019, journalist Sam Knight published a piece in *The New Yorker* on a psychiatrist's attempts to understand premonitions. He chronicles the work of English psychiatrist John

Barker, who in the mid-twentieth century became interested in what he called "pre-disaster syndrome," in which "'human seismographs' have bodily sensations ahead of important or emotional events." Knight recounts Barker's efforts to study these events within the realm of science, with systematic methodology. But unsurprisingly, despite having collected a remarkable set of examples in which premonitions bore out, sometimes tragically, there was no clear explanation for these events. In Knight's words, "Premonitions are impossible, and they come true all the time."

No matter what we believe about the origin point of gut instincts like these, what can we do with them? I know that my gut is good, that it is powerful. I know that it tends to warn me, to steer me away from situations that I am soon glad to have avoided, like car accidents. But the rightness of my gut can scare me. My gut has also been right when I wish it hadn't been—when I've anticipated something awful, and it's come to be true. When my beloved friend was diagnosed with a terminal illness. When it came to my dad's memory loss. Sometimes I think that it might have been better to be free of the accompanying anxiety for a little while longer, knowing that there was nothing I could do to change the future. In these instances, my gut seems to terrorize me, to egg on my anxiety, to bring about a sort of preemptive grief. I feel a physical change in myself, a sinking of the stomach, a clenching of the jaw. But also—these events loom large in my memory because they've been pivotal in my life. And I see that maybe I'm falling prey to that fallacy of remembering, even tallying, the exceptional situations instead of all the far more mundane moments in which my anxiety conjured disasters that never came to pass.

ℰ

How do we decide what to do, how to be? How do we determine which risks are worth taking, and which are best avoided? It's easy to say that we make decisions rationally, by undergoing a thorough, systematic process of risk-benefit analysis. That we think, with our brains, about the pros and cons that each move could bring about, and in this way, we come to well-thought-through decisions. But our decisions are impacted by forces and biases that are pragmatic and emotional, social and personal. We tend to view our decision-making as more logical than it actually is. Even in the best of times, we are not, as humans, particularly rational. For most of us, as we face large and small decisions, anxiety holds some degree of sway. That anxiety is part of the decision-making process isn't irrational or problematic in and of itself—in fact, a dose of anxiety is protective insofar as it protects us from recklessness. In excess, though, anxiety can get in the way of thinking through risks and making decisions. One might, for instance, choose to take a medication that carries some risk of side effects because research suggests that the benefits are likely to outweigh the risks. But this decision may prove unduly difficult, with the risks looming larger than data suggests that they should. Small print may be read a few times too many. Jokes may be made about how one could have become a lawyer, or maybe a pharmacist.

New parenthood is, for many people, a period of high anxiety alongside frequent and unavoidable decision-making. This anxiety has a form of its own—not only because it is an altogether new terrain with (accurately perceived) vast responsibility, but because also it is steeped in love. In this way, new parents, even those who are unaccustomed to anxiety, are faced with fears of mortality and of loss. Emily Oster, PhD, is a professor of economics at Brown University and a prolific writer whose work centers around pregnancy and parenthood—and in some circles, she has become a household name. Oster's work addresses issues like sleep training, feeding methods, and recently, COVID-19 safety, all from a data-driven perspective. And Oster's work also tends to interface directly with our bodies. Much of the data she discusses has to do with bodily health and safety in pregnancy, and decision-making about the well-being of pregnant people and young children. Thousands of parents look to Oster to temper their worries and find relief in her definitive tone and even-tempered use of data to make sense of parenting uncertainties. I cling to her statements, and I am certainly not alone— many times, I've heard friends say, "It's fine. Emily says it is." It can be a relief to leave it to someone else to decide, someone who knows more.

Oster's work raises questions about how we interface with data— that is, with capital-I Information—and how we make decisions. On one hand, in our current age, data feels infinitely available—yet so few of us know what to make of it. And even if we all had Oster's statistical expertise, I suspect that we would nonetheless look to someone else to help us make sense of what to do with it. We are still stuck with wondering what we can know and what we can be sure of, which is to say, how to decide which risks to take.

Oster taps into the experience of decision-making not just when we are anxious but when loss would be utterly devastating. When Oster shares data, that, for instance, pregnant people can safely eat sushi, she is actually alleviating fears that extend far beyond parasites. These are fears of being, for instance, a selfish, destructive person or a toxic mother. Risk perception and decision-making are never just about the thing in front of you. After all, we aren't computers, no matter how hard we sometimes try to be. Reading Oster can feel like someone has finally taken the weight of these decisions on, as though she's offered to carry it for you, with calm, direct reassurance.

Oster looks deeply at the issues that she writes about, and she gathers and synthesizes information—but also she recognizes that in the end, there are many things that we can't know for sure. Even more than I'm impressed by the data and the perspective that Oster offers, I wonder how she does it. What would it be like to have a mind like Oster's? How would it feel to walk through life able to look at the numbers, to understand them, to fully appreciate their merits and their imperfections, and then to get on with the day? How does one learn to live with it?

I talked to Oster about the particular ways that her work quells her readers' anxieties. She has a crystal-clear understanding of this dynamic, about the ways that by offering some clarity around concrete matters like whether to sleep train a one-year-old, we're really getting at far less concrete concerns, which she describes to me as "how to live with the ultimate uncertainty that we aren't equipped to tolerate." Oster knows that we have a tendency to focus on the parts of our lives that seem to be within the realm of our control.

We go on to talk about Oster's interest in helping parents learn to make decisions well. So often, people make decisions out of anxiety or fear, with a sense of urgency, or clouded with avoidance, and later live to regret it. Oster explains that when we make decisions based

on the best data that is available, we reduce the risk of negative outcomes, but also we gain some assurance that our decision was one
that came from a sound, thoughtful place, even if things don't go as
we had hoped.

Oster reminds us that no matter our attempts to be rational, and
despite the systems that exist to reduce risk, more often than not
we face decisions around which data is imperfect or unavailable. As
much as we wish that they were, right and wrong are not always so
easily cleaved. To be clear, I'm not suggesting that we should go
about our lives making decisions solely based on instinct, without
taking into account the information that is available to us, or past
experiences, or the wisdom of other people—but rather, that even
then, so much is, in the end, up to interpretation. We can take an
honest look at our decision-making processes, but then all that remains is to accept that no matter our best efforts, things may go off
the rails.

People who experience anxiety tend to perceive the risk of negative outcomes as greater compared with people who don't experience
anxiety. Do you drive over the speed limit? Eat the food that sat in
the fridge, with the door accidentally ajar, overnight? This sort of
seemingly minor matter can expose vast differences in the ways we
live. More than they reflect beliefs about driving or food safety, they
expose the varying degrees to which each of us feels at risk of harm
in the world. I drive the speed limit. A refrigerator door left open
strikes me as a hearty welcome to food poisoning. Whenever I see a
painting that includes a skull or any other kind of memento mori, I
wonder how it is possible that anyone needs to be reminded that
death comes for us all.

Anxiety can sway decision-making in other ways too. The affect heuristic, a common bias in decision-making, is defined as "reliance on affect in situations of risk and uncertainty." The affect heuristic is at work when our feelings unduly sway our decisions. These feelings can be positive or negative—say, excitement about a new job opportunity or anxiety about your child spending the night away from home. Our emotional state can override other important sources of information.

Anxiety is associated with a tendency to make considerable efforts to avoid feared outcomes, even when there is potential for reward. In our daily lives, what might rewards entail? Stepping out of the confines of clinical research, when we make decisions, conscious of it or not, we are often facing these very issues. It might be something small—say, will I introduce myself to this person who could become a friend, or is the risk of rejection too great? Or something with obvious repercussions—will I apply for a better job, knowing that I may not get it? All of which is to say, can I tolerate risk if reward is possible? When we are led about by our anxiety, life can feel small.

The differences in each of our perceptions of risk have never been so front and center as during the COVID-19 pandemic. Some of us saw COVID-19 as more risky than others, and you'd be hard-pressed to find a person who didn't experience some degree of conflict, whether with friends or family or colleagues, over these differences. In my family, as I suspect is true for most all of us, we spanned the full spectrum of responses. Some of us spent a great deal of time at home, tested often, constantly masked in public, and were vaccinated as soon as we could be, whereas others went about their lives without much concern. There were the worriers and the care-free, and there was little movement between camps. The conflicts that emerged between us were not small, not easily resolved—because in the end, it was always about more than COVID-19. When you make decisions about risk, you are making decisions about how to live, and these are choices that weigh differently on each of us.

Beyond family conflict, the COVID-19 pandemic created the conditions for research that might otherwise have been relegated to thought experiments or laboratory manipulations. In a study that was conducted in mid-2020, researchers in Nigeria looked at the relationship between anxiety levels and risk perception in the context of the pandemic and found that the risks of COVID-19 seemed greater to those with higher levels of anxiety. Another study, conducted in Italy during the first year of the pandemic, also found a link between perceptions of greater risk and higher levels of anxiety.

During periods of the pandemic in which I felt risk to be greatest, especially when case counts were high near my home, I felt most anxious when I feared that I had inadvertently exposed someone to COVID-19. I held my breath until (more than) enough days had passed that it seemed nobody had become ill, at least not with me as the disease vector. Rather than viewing these periods of time as one of many inevitable, awful aspects of a pandemic, no matter our best intentions, I felt like an accidental agent of destruction (and remember, nobody had actually become sick). Anxiety distorts the ways we think about risk prevention. Despite knowing better, when we're anxious, we more easily fall prey to the idea that it is possible to assess risk perfectly and to control risk completely. But if what you need to find peace of mind is total certainty, you'll be waiting forever.

"Control" is a tricky term—and it carries with it a good deal of negative and positive connotations. We tend to associate control with keeping a tight grip on things—with attempting to dictate the movements of other people, for instance, or to prevent the unpreventable. But there is another kind of control, one that has to do instead with the way we feel within ourselves, and the degree to which we feel a sense of power in the world. This, to me, is about agency. It is about feeling that we are not simply at the whim of the world, but rather we are actors in it. Researchers have, for decades, looked at the ways in which we experience control. Where do we feel that control comes from? To what degree do we feel that we can dictate the goings-on in our own lives, and to what degree do we feel we are at the mercy of the world around us? And what does this mean for our well-being? A great deal of psychological research suggests that people who experience anxiety (and also depression) are prone to feeling a lack of control from within themselves. Rather, they tend to feel that their life experiences are dictated by other people or forces. This stance is known as an external locus of control. On the other hand, those with an internal locus of control generally feel a sense of agency in the world—as though they have power, control over their own lives. They feel that they can make things happen, or make them not happen—and this is associated with well-being. Our sense of where control comes from seems to be long-lasting (in fact, one study found locus of control to be consistent over nearly a decade, despite inevitable changes in participants' lives).

We see anxiety tied to an external locus of control time and time again—and this makes intuitive sense. None of us wants to feel powerless. But I find, too, that I'm left with lingering questions. For as much as anxiety gets kicked up when we feel out of control, anxiety can sometimes bring with it feelings of too much control—too much power. When we're anxious, control, power—they seem to double over on themselves. We talk a lot about the ways that anxiety can reflect our desperation to hold on to control. But what if we fear our own control too? What if we perceive our potential for control as dangerous, overwhelming? This is where responsibility comes in.

Do you like to be responsible, in control, to be the one who decides things? Or does the weight of responsibility weigh heavily on you, more heavily than it seems to weigh on most other people? Do you tend to feel as though you are highly responsible but lack control? These are questions more easily asked than answered. Anxiety exposes the complexities and paradoxes that shape each of our relationships to responsibility and control. I find over and over that the two move together; they can't be entirely separated from each other. Our sense of being responsible influences our feelings about control. Since the 1980s, researchers and clinicians have been studying the ways in which people with obsessive-compulsive disorder (OCD) experience responsibility, from both theoretical and experimental perspectives. It has since been well established that OCD is associated with an inflated sense of responsibility. For people with OCD, the weight of responsibility can feel terribly heavy, and it can extend great distances. I think again of the term "tender conscience," first used, as you recall, to (tenderly!) describe OCD by Stanley Rachman. Research shows that an inflated, even overwhelming sense of responsibility isn't unique to OCD—it can be symptomatic of other forms of anxiety, too, like generalized anxiety disorder (GAD). It bears repeating that anxiety disorders are more often diagnosed in women than in men—and, too, when it comes to GAD, an inflated sense of responsibility may also be more common in women than in men. While some research addresses the biological factors that may be at play, it strikes me that these disparities are also reflective of long-standing societal inequities. Women are often socialized to silently shoulder the burden of responsibility for other people, practically and emotionally. Eventually, the rubber has to meet the road.

Imagine that you are walking down a hallway in your office building. You are late for a meeting. Then, out of the corner of your eye, you see a drop of water on the floor. You think to yourself that if you don't get a paper towel to clean up the drop of water and someone slips on it and hits their head and subsequently dies, their death will rest on your shoulders. It will have been your fault. You will have been responsible. So you turn around, find a bathroom, get a paper towel, and crouch on the floor of the hallway to make sure that the water is well and truly gone. You are late for your meeting, but your mind is, at least momentarily, at ease.

Anxiety evokes the feeling that if one is careful enough, responsible enough, attentive enough to every possible outcome—essentially, worried enough—it might be possible to ward off devastation. But hypervigilance will never achieve what we wish it could—it cannot preclude disaster or mortality. None of us is so powerful.

In our own ways and at our own times, we all face questions about risk, about responsibility, and about agency. Most of us are trying to sort out how to be, no matter our age or position in life. How do I want to be, how do most of us want to be? We want to be able to take risks, with consideration and to a point. To make decisions based on the information that is available, and then to move on. To have power over our own lives, to have some control, but not too much. To go about life responsibly, within reason. To live, as much as possible, according to our most deeply felt values and instincts, strengthened by the courage that is always within. To follow meaning, curiosity, and love. Which is to say, to be led by the gut. Just as there are consequences to ignoring one's guts, there is joy in following them. There is a thrill in "no." The pleasure of defiance, that most potent antidote to anxiety, that is the pleasure of the gut.

Over time, you feel acquiescence in your gut. It eats at you, like an ulcer. It builds resentment and anger, and in the long term, it increases anxiety. To counteract this pattern requires constant, active practice. It requires facing one's own beliefs, taking ownership of them, and accepting the fallout, whatever it may be. It may never feel automatic or natural, but defiance can be learned, and defiance is what allows you to stand firm even in the face of the worst anxiety. When I think of the times when I've exercised my gut in spite of my anxiety—when I've, for instance, advocated for myself in difficult circumstances—I find that in the days that follow, I feel a sort of high. I feel quietly brave, empowered by the strength that I myself have generated. When I've acted fully in accordance with my gut—not in anxiety's absence, but in its presence—this is agency. This is guts.

When I was a child, I collected quotations. I would cut them out of magazines and write them down in notebooks. My maternal grandmother, an Italian American woman born in 1922 who was warm and loving and truly fabulous, always beautifully dressed, bejeweled, and perfumed, got into doing this with me. Her sources were far-reaching, but mostly she was drawn to self-help. She recorded quotes from Pope Francis. From *O, The Oprah Magazine*, and *Real Simple*. From Al-Anon books. Even Pilates guides. When I graduated from high school, she presented me with a book of quotations that she had collected for me over the years—with entries like "Nothing is impossible. The word itself says 'I'm Possible!'" (Audrey Hepburn) and "Be yourself; everybody else is already taken" (Oscar Wilde), written with her signature purple uni-ball pen, in her gorgeous script.

My grandmother had a way of noticing when I was trying to spit something out, struggling to muster up the courage to say aloud what I really thought. Decades later, I see that she knew this struggle intimately, and I see the tragedy in it. Like many women of her generation, she held so much back. She acquiesced and shuttered away the things that gnawed at her, and the consequences ran deep. Much remained unsaid, and I suspect she suffered for it. When she was in her last years, we'd speak on the phone a few times a week. Often I had the feeling that something was on her mind, and I would urge her to tell me what was troubling her, to get the words out of her. But our conversations would end with the verbal equivalent of a knowing glance.

When we're wrestling with a problem in our own lives, words or phrases stand out to us in ways they wouldn't otherwise. Something we hear feels particularly wise, particularly elegant or to the point, or its meaning strikes us anew. At a time when I was struggling to advocate for myself, and, I see now, struggling to act in accordance with my gut (struggling to acknowledge my gut at all), a mentor of mine said to another student: "You know, you may have to take shit, but you don't have to eat it." Although I was only witness to them, his words felt as though they were meant especially for me.

We have no choice but to live amid societal pressures and conditions that we wouldn't choose. No matter the degree to which anxiety influences our lives, all of us are subject to being swayed by our surroundings and to the particular complexities of our own histories. But it is for us to notice, and to pay close attention, and then to act, when the forces that drown out our guts exceed that innermost sense. When it comes to reaching the body, reaching the gut, words tend to fall short. Instead, we are moved beyond language by a piece of music, or by the astounding beauty of the natural world, or by human touch. We all have our leanings—I rely heavily on words. The fact is, I love them. I always have, and I suspect I always will. But just as we can look inward to find better words, to articulate our experiences with more clarity, understanding comes in many forms. Sometimes, it hovers over language, somewhere in the gut.

I don't keep a book of quotations anymore, but I do keep a tiny notebook, maybe three inches long by two inches wide, of words that strike me for one reason or another, words I want to hold on to. Sometimes I forget about it for a while, and sometimes I reach for it twice in one day, but it's always sitting on my desk. I've been doing this for years, and though I've never dated the entries, they evoke different points in my life. Beset by. Ensnare. Interstitial. Redrawn. Metabolize. Incorporate. Insistent. Muscular. Incantatory. I feel them, echoing, in my gut.

Part V

POSSIBILITIES

9.

SUBLIMATION
AND SUBVERSION

Inside the word *emergency* is *emerge*;
from an emergency new things come forth.
The old certainties are crumbling fast,
but danger and possibility are sisters.

—Rebecca Solnit, *Hope in the Dark*

I'm texting with a friend, another psychologist, and I miss a pop culture reference, something to do with a chef. I tell her that I think I am living under a rock. She responds:

> Stay under that rock
> The world is trash.

She is kidding, sort of. She is actually one of the more hopeful, buoyant people I know. But then, the undercurrent is always there. Is every wall really a door?

Anxiety is often framed as a survival mechanism. But anxiety has other meanings too. When we are anxious, we are reminded that there is so much we cannot know, and that cause and effect are imperfectly related—after all, we are not machines. Anxiety is an attempt, and a painful one at that, to face the world and to solve the unsolvable. It asks those big questions that are inherent to our lives: What will happen to us? How much change is possible? These are questions that are not only for those whose anxiety meets criteria for a diagnosis—they are for all of us, and they will always be a part of human life.

Science can be a double-edged sword. On one hand, it is among our greatest teachers—it presents us with opportunities to understand ourselves and one another that would have been impossible even a few years ago. But somehow, the more we come to know, the more tightly we seem to grip the knowledge that we do have as unchangeable. To make matters more difficult, currently available scientific methodologies lend themselves to identifying definable, often short-term treatments, and they can fail to capture the messy reality of our lives. In this way, we can fall prey to an illusion of certainty that backfires. It leads us to think that we know far more than we do, and we close our minds to possibility. The scientists, artists, and thinkers who go down in history for having been far ahead of their time, the ones whose work was met with resistance if not persecution, recognized that we were (are, will always be!) only beginning to see the edges of things. But then, in this destabilization, there is, paradoxically, a kind of comfort. There is no use in holding certainty so tightly. In its place, we can access wonder, even awe. In the space between yearning for control and letting go, there are worlds, and there is possibility.

As a psychologist, I was trained to think about mental illness and mental health care in terms of a meeting point of factors, coming from within and outside our bodies. Yet I've found that treatment often fails to bring this meeting to a place of true fruition. Though medication and talk therapy often work in conjunction, there remains a disconnect in the ways that we think, and talk about, our experiences and our bodies. Our bodies transcend the realm of biology even in their physicality—and so does resilience.

We use a range of terms in psychological settings and in our daily lives to refer to ideas of resilience, with some being anchored more firmly in established definitions than others. And depending on whom you ask, you will hear a slightly different definition of resilience. Broadly speaking, resilience has to do with our capacity to weather hard times. The American Psychological Association defines resilience as "the process and outcome of successfully adapting to difficult or challenging life experiences, especially through mental, emotional, and behavioral flexibility, and adjustment to internal and external demands." I think again of my conversation with Stephen Porges about polyvagal theory, during which he made the point, with respect to heart rate, that "oscillation is healthy!" Flexibility fosters resilience from both physiological and emotional standpoints.

Some researchers delineate resilience and coping based on the severity of the situations that they are a response to, with the idea being that coping happens when we respond to minor struggles, whereas resilience is tested when we face larger ones. One might, for instance, demonstrate their coping skills (say, maintaining an exercise routine or sleeping at least seven hours per night) in the context of an unusually stressful month at work, whereas their resilience would be tested if they were to live through a natural disaster.

In economic terms, understanding resilience, and then, developing strategies to build and bolster it, are ways to offset the massive costs of anxiety, on both societal and individual levels. Resilience helps us to maintain, or to more quickly return to, our usual responsibilities. In more human terms, resilience is a kind of power in the face of the world. When we cultivate resilience within ourselves, hard times come to feel less like end times, because we carry with us a belief that above all, we will survive. Indeed, resilience protects us: Studies on resilience in the context of the COVID-19 pandemic abound. We know well that this was a time of historically high stress levels, especially for first responders. In June 2020, researchers in Europe conducted a study, with nurses as participants, to look at the ways in which resilience may impact the relationship between anxiety, depression, and stress. They found that higher scores on a measure of resilience were associated with fewer symptoms of anxiety and depression—that is, "resilience played a protective role." In the face of tragic circumstances, this study (and others like it) highlights the importance of resilience as a process that we should be attending to with care, a process that can, indeed, be a buffer. Resilience matters for all of us—for the anxious, for the not-so-anxious, for those who struggle with mental health in other respects, and even for those who do not. We are all subject to unexpected setbacks, to loss, to tragedy.

We can think of resilience through other lenses too. We ask, in so many words, can we make ourselves anew? This is a question that we will face forever. Human history is built on stories of rebirth, of spring, and of our attempts to transform one thing into another—into something, in essence, better. The alchemy of the Middle Ages asked, fundamentally, is change possible? And if it is, how much? We look to religious texts, or to ancient mythologies, or to literature. Across time and place, we see ourselves in these stories. We feel a bit less alone—and we see that sometimes, things do change. A phoenix rises from the ashes. A superhero who, as a child, suffers a tragic loss, returns, powerful. A scarab beetle brings the promise of a new day. In noticing when we feel ourselves seduced by the promise of trans-formation, we can, with our skepticism in hand, look inward. We can identify the parts of ourselves that we are struggling with and the strengths that we want so badly to develop.

We can look to the natural world, too, and then, within our own bodies (inseparable from the natural world whether we like it or not), to show us resilience. We see the cycles of the moon, or the changes in plant life over the course of a month, a year. We are hun-gry and then full. Asleep and awake and asleep again. Our brains undergo neuronal pruning, with some areas growing with age and others atrophying. Our world and our bodies are constantly facing beginnings, endings, and, sometimes, renewal.

In *Islands of Abandonment: Nature Rebounding in the Post-Human Landscape*, Cal Flyn describes resilience in the natural world, against all odds: "This is a corrupted world, yes—one long fallen from a state of grace—but it is a world too that knows how to live. It has a great capacity for repair, for recovery, for forgiveness—of a sort—if we can only learn to let it do so. Lands cleared for cultivation centuries before revert to forest in a matter of years. Environments stripped of their inhabitants can repopulate of their own accord. Even contaminated sites of the very worst kind can, when given the chance, become ecosystems of singular importance." Hope and dread. We see the coming together of disaster and rebuilding, of struggle and potential. We see, too, that change is inevitable, that, as so many wisdom traditions teach us, nothing, and certainly no feeling, is permanent. It turns out that we, too, are capable of remarkable change. Mere mortals, we struggle, we learn, we try again. But in this persistence, this daily insistence, there can be integrity.

My son tells me that he saw a video on YouTube about how hamsters gnaw off their own limbs if they get injured. He tells me that after they gnaw them off, the limbs regrow, like the limbs of a chameleon. They can, he explains, have new arms and new legs. He wants me to search YouTube for a video of their limbs regrowing. I tell him I don't think this is possible for hamsters, that there must be some confusion, let's not look it up—and that not all creatures can do this. But he insists that it is possible, that, in fact, there is a special enzyme.

ॐ

Although so much of our well-being can feel predetermined, whether by genetics or environmental exposures, we do ourselves a disservice if we lose sight of our own potential for change. Resilience is a way of being that we can cultivate. We can develop our resilience through engaging in certain practices and experiences—like mindfulness and psychotherapy—and by developing our capacity for flexibility and our distress tolerance and emotion regulation skills. And we can develop resilience in communion with one another.

Though we tend to view resilience and coping as individual pursuits (we wonder what it is about a person's personality that seems to make them resilient, for instance), resilience is a multidimensional process that develops within *and* between people—not in isolation. Research consistently finds that while there seem to be aspects of our personalities and biology that do indeed support resilience, resilience is not simply a set of personality characteristics that you have or don't have. Instead, resilience is a matter of the experiences we have, throughout our lives, within systems that extend far beyond ourselves and, too, beyond our individual control. In this spirit, here is another, systems-based definition of resilience from psychologist and resilience expert Ann S. Masten: "Resilience can be broadly defined as the capacity of a dynamic system to adapt successfully to disturbances that threaten system function, viability, or development. The concept can be applied to systems of many kinds at many interacting levels, both living and nonliving, such as a microorganism, a child, a family, a security system, an economy, a forest, or the global climate."

When we think about the body and its capacity for change and resilience, we need to look outside the standard boundaries of health care, to history, to economics, to sociology, to policymaking. Children learn about resilience from their caregivers. They witness the ways in which their caregivers get through difficult times, for better and for worse. But also they see the ways that communities and social systems support people, or don't. When we think about cultivating resilience, we should be thinking, alongside our biology, of the ways that we support one another. We should be attending to the structures that foster resilience—families, yes, but also communities and societies in which well-being is meaningfully supported—in which we mutually care for one another.

In recent history, we've lost many of the structures that once provided a degree of relief from anxiety. We used to go through life surrounded by communities that framed the unknown and taught us how to face it—often through ritual and religious practice. Terrible things were assumed to happen, they were an undeniable part of life, rather than relegated to "unlikely." And though varying forms of predestination and omniscience did not in any sense eliminate suffering, they did provide a structure through which to view life and death, and usually, people to do it with. Today's emphasis on reason is not especially conducive to ritual or to community building. After all, it is hard to worship logic.

We see that rituals hold us up as individuals and as communities—and that we use rituals to soothe ourselves and to bond with one another. They can be a way toward resilience. Rituals are woven throughout our lives, in small moments and at times of transition, celebration, and loss. Rituals bond communities, and they imbue the passage of time with meaning. They give structure to our internal lives, and they soothe loneliness. Children love rituals—and we see that they thrive within them. School begins with the same song each day. Friday night is movie night. Before bedtime comes bath time and stories. As adults, we repeat some of the rituals that we were raised with, and over time we create our own. These are often simple acts, but they aren't trivial. They remind us that despite so much uncertainty, despite our inevitable struggles, despite our fears and our worries, time moves forward, and we aren't alone in it.

It turns out that in addition to reducing anxiety levels, rituals can improve other aspects of our well-being. In a recent study conducted in England, researchers looked at how secular rituals and religious ones, which included some of the same structures, compared. People attended either communal religious gatherings or communal secular gatherings, and in both cases, they felt more bonded with one another and more emotional positivity after participating. We understand on an intuitive level, too, that rituals are one of the ways that we soothe ourselves—that we reach for rituals in stressful times. Anxiety, ever the opportunistic affliction, seems to emerge and expand in the space that lost rituals leave behind. I think of the early days of the COVID-19 pandemic, a time of unprecedented global anxiety and radical loss of ritual. People around the world began to have regular Zoom gatherings with friends whom they would otherwise have seen regularly in person. There were virtual book clubs, virtual birthday parties. The underwhelming and often melancholy virtual holidays. We would have "virtual pub night" with a close friend, sitting in our quiet living room while he sat in his, and though it wasn't the same, it reminded us that we were connected. The loss of ritual was deeply destabilizing, and many of us looked for substitutions.

We see the importance of being in communion with other people in mental health care too. The sine qua non of psychotherapy, no matter the school of thought to which you belong, is that people are capable of change. Research on the psychotherapy process has, for decades, tried to identify the change agents, the driving forces of change in treatment. What does change hinge on? What is it that really helps? Is it, for instance, the particular type of psychotherapy

that you participate in? Or is it the presence or absence of psychotherapy homework? Or, perhaps, the length of treatment? Time and
time again, research finds that, in fact, one of the central aspects of
change in psychotherapy is the relationship that exists between the
patient and the therapist, known as the therapeutic alliance. Fundamentally, it is in meaningful interactions with another person, in
connection itself, that we seem to find our way. I think again of
Porges's polyvagal theory, and the ways in which it emphasizes the
importance of connecting, with a sense of safety, with other people.
Porges writes, "Resiliency might be a product of a nervous system
with sufficient resources to move out of the self-oriented focus of
threat and stress to an other-oriented focus of feelings of safety that
naturally emerge into actions of sociality, and compassion." This
would be the ultimate therapeutic outcome.

I asked Porges how he thinks about resilience in the context of
polyvagal theory, and especially the principle that resilience happens
with other people, rather than in isolation. He said, "If we claim our
evolutionary heritage, which is to connect with others, who do we
become?" I hear this, and I feel a wave of hope, a wave of optimism
in the face of so much chaos. Well-being, meaning, even resilience
itself—they all emerge out of caring for one another.

Resilience and change can't be reduced to formulas—they require
imagination. They are the building and rebuilding of ourselves.
They aren't done once and then complete—rather, we are in perpetual states of reshaping. And although we are drawn, like moths to a
flame, to tangible, concrete outcomes, internal change is often only
roughly quantified or altogether intangible. To be resilient is to be
elastic, to be flexible, to be able to tolerate changes, pushes and pulls,

without snapping. Our systems of understanding need to be resilient too—which is to say, we need resilience, flexibility, capacity for change and recovery—in the ways we think about mental health, and in the ways we approach studying it.

There are forms of change, and maybe, forms of resilience, that we are only beginning to understand. Placebo effects are often written off as "fake" change, or as results that are all in one's head, so to speak. In a remarkable study on the placebo effect as it relates to physical exercise, researchers followed a group of people who worked in housekeeping at a hotel over the course of one month. They told half of the participants that their work constituted exercise, whereas they didn't provide any such explanation to the other half of the participants. Despite the fact that all the participants continued to work as usual, those who had been told that their work was a form of exercise had improved physical health at the end of the study period. Placebo effects raise questions about how we may be able to effect change within our own bodies, and about the place of belief and hope in our susceptibility to change. When it comes to treatment for anxiety disorders (and depression), placebo response rates to some medications have been a source of ongoing controversy as they can be especially high. Scientists are learning more about the factors that underly placebo effects, and their findings are staggering.

The placebome, a term coined by molecular biologist Dr. Kathryn T. Hall, is "the hypothesized group of genome related or derived molecules . . . that affect an individual's response to placebo treatment." Hall's research points toward genetic markers that could explain why some people respond to placebos, while others do not. That is, it may be that some people's genetics make them more likely to respond to placebos than other people. Research on the placebome could open the door to new questions and new lines of research when it comes to resilience. I wonder—do those who respond to the placebo effect have an internal mechanism for recovery, and perhaps resilience? And again, I feel hopeful and curious. Work on the placebome could turn existing research on its head by calling into question the ways in which we've traditionally interpreted placebo responses, and the ways that clinical trials are designed. I spoke to Hall about her research, and we talked about the factors at play in the placebome, and, too, about another component of placebo effects known as placebogenic providers—a term that refers to the ways in which certain health-care providers, whether therapists or nurses or doctors, may have more positive impact on their patients than other providers. This is not only a matter of bedside manner, though that is certainly important—it is a matter of equity in health care. In a paper coauthored by Hall and colleagues, they explain:

> While positive expectations can produce beneficial effects, negative information and experiences can lead to negative expectations, and consequently negative or nocebo effects. Key components identified and studied in the placebo and nocebo literature intersect with factors identified as barriers to quality care in the clinical setting for Black patients and other patients of color. . . . in the context of discrimination and bias, the absence of placebo and presence of nocebo-generating influences in clinical settings could potentially reinforce racial and ethnic inequalities in clinical outcomes and care.

Whether in psychotherapy or in medical settings or elsewhere, we see over and over that health, recovery, and resilience do not exist in a vacuum. They are shaped, inevitably, by the systems we operate within, and by the ways in which we care for one another.

&

When I get even the smallest of injuries, my body takes weeks to heal. This has always been true of me—I have scars from minor childhood accidents, the kind that are altogether unremarkable but memorable to me only because the scars remain. A scraped knee on a driveway, or a fall off a bicycle thirty-some years ago. I find that my easy scarring mirrors an internal sensitivity too. My emotional wounds remain for longer than I would like. I find them difficult to shake off, and the worry or sadness that accompanies them stays with me. When I was a child, my mother used to tell me, with the sort of empathy that comes from personal experience, that I needed to learn to have thicker skin. I was too permeable to these small injuries—my feelings were hurt so easily. I would pinch the outer surfaces of my hands to show her just how thin my skin seemed to be. In retrospect, I see that what I was wrestling with was more than an elusive toughness—it was that I wanted to learn to be resilient.

I see now that anxiety brings with it all sorts of sensitivity. Just as it heightens awareness of our own internal bodily sensations, it impacts our experiences of other people, and of the world too. Sometimes, perhaps against my better judgment, I still wish that I had thicker skin. I wish that I were, somehow, unflappable. I wonder if I could change myself in this way, once and for all. I imagine what it would be like to develop an internal resistance, a protective membrane that would be impermeable to fear and worry and dread. But then, we can't have it both ways. Impermeability fosters isolation, not connection. So instead I try to think of resilience. I remind myself that resilience is a constant practice rather than a discrete outcome—and it can give anxiety a new shape. And I remember that anxiety is potential, it is a force, one that can become something else. I remember, too, that I don't have to like my anxieties, but I do have to live with them—and that it is in the living that I take my power back. And this feels like a taste of magic, in human form.

As a wise teacher once told me, you have to get up and you have to put on your shoes. In its most literal interpretation, you could argue that this is a behavioral approach. That, even when you feel anxious (or depressed, or any number of other things), you need to do the thing you don't feel like doing in order to change how you feel. This approach aligns with cognitive behavioral therapy in that it presupposes that your feelings will follow your behaviors—not the other way around. Instead of staying in bed, you take a shower. Instead of canceling social plans, you go out. You look to your behaviors to shape how you feel, instead of looking for your feelings to shape your behaviors. These behavioral strategies can be a powerful way to begin to treat anxiety. But in my experience, it is equally important to provide another frame for these techniques. They are more than a behavioral intervention, and they are more than just "pushing through." Getting up, putting on one's proverbial shoes, this isn't only a technique to reduce the discomfort that anxiety brings with it—it can also be the beginnings of a new way of relating to anxiety and a new way of understanding it. By forging ahead in spite of, even alongside anxiety, you put it in its place. Anxiety tempts us inward, but it can also be propulsive. In the words of Samuel Beckett: "I can't go on. I'll go on." Everything is in the going on. All is not lost, but some things will be. Many things are possible. This is, perhaps, the essence of resilience.

So we see that, in body and in mind, we are remarkably resilient. Our brains are plastic. Our thoughts are plastic. Our nervous systems, our cardiovascular systems, our microbiomes, even our blood— all possess a remarkable capacity for change. But equally, the real changes that we are after, and the sort that we are capable of, aren't responsive to quick fixes. Change depends on our communities, our systems, the worlds outside of us—we are not, in the end, islands. And sometimes, even then, even with the pieces in place, we are what we are. Even with so much potential for change in the body, there is nonetheless some heartbreak. When we think about plasticity, we face its edges and limits. There are surely forms of plasticity, forms of potential, forms of change, that we have yet to conceptualize, yet to have any sense of at all. After all, in the scheme of things, it was not so long ago that humans came to understand DNA or penicillin or even the cells that make up our bodies. Even within limits, hope remains. Hope and dread, hope and dread. Anxiety reminds us that there is perpetual friction between the two, and that we can't look away. We can be insistent in our hopefulness without discounting the uncertainties and the tragedies that life contains—and we can, with time, learn to live amid these forces with a sense of meaning. We can experience awe at all that is possible, in our bodies and in the world, in all their imperfection.

We are far from solving the problems of anxiety. But we do have beginnings, and we have big ideas. As is so often the case, it seems that we have more clarity about the problem than about how to fix it—more questions than answers. The same is true within ourselves. Too often, emotional change is thought of in completist terms. We are cured, or we aren't. All has been achieved, or all is lost. Rather than seeing our struggles in terms of waves of change, constantly shifting, we look through the lenses of progress and decline—and we forget that emotional change isn't linear. We are, as a collective, facing the limits of these modes of thinking—and we are seeing the beginnings of new, more creative, and more flexible frameworks for thinking about change, about self-improvement, and about what re-silience really means. In this way, we are finding that anxiety is an experience that exists within and outside of ourselves—that is, anxi-ety exists in the meeting of ourselves and the world.

I'm anxious about my upcoming deadline. My husband texts me, en-couragingly: "as long as panic is being channeled into fire you're good!" This will always be my work. Sigmund Freud wrote about sublima-tion, a process by which, in response to urges and impulses we have that we feel are unacceptable, we do something else that does feel ac-ceptable, even useful. Through this lens, the process of sublimation, of coming to redirect one's energy for good, was tied to the most central facets of human experience—"art, science, philosophy, religion, and civilization itself," as described in the tome *Psychoanalytic Terms and Concepts*. In fact, sublimation was categorized as being among the most mature, adaptive defense mechanisms available to us.

Now, when I think about sublimation, I think of the many ways that all of us are trying, day in and day out, to change one thing into another, to transform aspects of ourselves and our lives. We look for the growth that can come out of a difficult experience, or for the beginning that can come from a painful end. I think of transforming anxiety—of putting it to good use, making it into power. And I like to think, then, about the word "subversion"—because it connotes change alongside defiance. In the *Oxford English Dictionary*, definitions of subversion include: "The overturning . . . of an established or existing practice; The transformation of a state of things; the action of upsetting or overturning a thing." To transform anxiety into a force of one's own—to subvert it—it's a kind of rebellion.

So, when anxiety beckons, will I snarl back?

We study resilience. We try to identify its causes and effects, to name and measure the factors that strengthen it. But there is another kind of resilience, too, in recognizing that even amid the unmeasurables and unknowns, of which there are so very many, we can have hope. That things can change, we can change. Not completely, but often, enough. Ruth Ozeki, the writer and Zen Buddhist priest, has described "the generative tension between knowing and not knowing." Anxiety generates this sort of tension—between knowing and not knowing, between wanting to know and tolerating uncertainty. In this tension, there is anxiety, but tension itself can birth something new. In the newness, there is resilience.

Our bodies are resilient, they can recover from grave injury. Our wounds can heal, if imperfectly. Our blood regenerates. We can, to a point, train our hearts to work more efficiently, to be more powerful. Our guts shift in accordance with the foods and medicines that they are exposed to, and even in accordance with our feelings. Our bodies are worlds of their own, constantly changing, sometimes within the bounds of our control, but often not. There are worlds within and outside of ourselves—worlds overlapping, interacting, in constant communication.

There are some psychological schools of thought that argue that anxiety (or, say, depression) isn't so much a part of oneself as it is an experience that people live with, that we struggle with. In this way, we can learn to separate our feelings from our identity. This approach can be helpful, this placing of anxiety outside ourselves, because it can create space for other experiences, and more so, for a larger sense of oneself, one that extends beyond painful symptoms. But. I find that, when I'm most honest with myself, I see that anxiety is indeed part of me, part of my identity. Not all of me, but part of me—and I know that I am in good company. There is no unbothered "me" beneath it. Rather, anxiety shapes us, just like other qualities—those that we enjoy or at least don't suffer from—do. Energy is lost to so many places in the course of a life, and for many, it is lost to anxiety. When we come to see the ways in which our pain shapes us, we can say something like, "That thought, that thought is just my anxiety"—but we can also say, "It is still mine." It can be mine, part of me, without being all of me. My anxiety shapes me, but so does my attention, my curiosity, my perseverance, my resistance, so does my joy. I find that in accepting that anxiety is within me, I am less often at war with it. I can see that it is there, in my organs, in my cells, in my thoughts, but I know that it will not subsume me.

Sometimes, we find our answers in our problems. Our bodies remind us of our fragility, and, ultimately, of our mortality. But also, they teach us. There is a multidimensional language of the body, if only we choose to listen to it, one that is shaped by external and internal forces. It is a language that is made up of words, sometimes, and also of feelings and sensations. In this way, words give form to our bodily experiences—they contain our bodies—and our bodies contain our words. We are carnal vessels, and so much more. Despite the uncertainty that surrounds us, and despite the anxiety that comes with seeing it, there is far more that is possible than the facts in front of us, than the surface that stares us down. There is reality, too, in the depth and wonder and mystery and unknowability of our lives. This is why when I think about anxiety, I have to think of more— this is my imperative. I think about anxiety, and then I think about boundaries, about truth. I think of limits and edges, of ambivalences. I think of our bodies—our brains, our hearts, our blood, our guts— which is to say, I think about attention and curiosity, about love, about the worlds within us all. Janus-like, I look back and I look forward. I think about depth and history, and always, perseverance. I summon the words, the fire, I summon the body.

Acknowledgments

My wholehearted thanks go first to Emma Finn, without whom this book quite simply would not exist. Brilliant, perceptive, and full of warmth, Emma understood this book—and, really, understood me—from the start. I also want to express my immense gratitude to the C&W translation rights team: Kate Burton, César Castañeda Gámez, Sam Downs, and Polly Peraza-Brown.

I am deeply grateful to Emily Wunderlich and Anna Steadman for their astute insights, thoughtfulness, precision, and devotion to this project, and for seeing the shape of this book from the beginning; and my thanks also go to their wonderful teams at Viking and Headline Home.

Thank you to my mentors and supervisors over the years—especially Nicole Van Nortwick, PhD, and Mark Kuras, PhD, whose wisdom and kindness are unmatched. They know what depth is; they have shown me the way.

I want to thank the late Jeremy Safran, PhD, my first mentor in the field of psychology. Jeremy's encouragement, kindness, and high expectations made me feel that I could be a psychologist, and that I could write.

Thank you to the clinicians and researchers who talked with me for this book, who shared their time and their expertise, and whose insights were invaluable: Jonathan S. Abramowitz, PhD; Travis E. Gibson, PhD; Kathryn T. Hall, PhD, MPH; Cameron Norsworthy, PhD; Emily Oster, PhD; Stephen W. Porges, PhD; Lawrence H. Price, MD; Alexander Shackman, PhD; Shankar Tumati, MBBS, PhD; and Nur Hani Zainal, PhD.

Without wonderful childcare, I could not have written this book. My gratitude to the people who do this work cannot be over-stated.

I want to thank the people who saw value in this project from its inception. They generously read early drafts, and they encour-aged me: Ari Aster, Sam Hanson, and Noah Sacco. And my trusted friends and confidants, whose insights are unmatched, for their frankness, humor, and sensitivity. They made me laugh, they recommended books, they listened to my worries: Laura Bhatt, LCSW; Meredith Carlisle, LCSW; Robin Carolan; Aimee Mil-liken, PhD; Lia Okun, PhD; Ali Shames-Dawson, PhD; and Anya Taylor-Joy.

Thank you, finally, to my family, whose love and support is unwavering—especially my sister, Lily, who makes me laugh when nobody else can; my mother, Paula, for teaching me to see depth and to love books from the start; and my father, George, who has always understood, and who always has the right words.

And most of all to Rob, my other half, my home, who makes all things possible, and to Houston, the light of my life.

Notes

Author's Note

xiv **"the magic combination":** Maria Popova, *Figuring* (Edinburgh: Canongate Books, 2019), 428.

Anxiety and Me: Anxiety as Potential

2 **"The term 'anxiety'":** Barbara Cassin, Emily Apter, Jacques Lezra, and Michael Wood, eds., *Dictionary of Untranslatables* (Princeton, NJ: Princeton University Press, 2014).

6 **Carl Jung wrote:** Carl Gustav Jung, *On the Nature of the Psyche* (New York: Routledge Classics, 2001).

10 **"palpitation of the heart":** Robert Burton, *The Anatomy of Melancholy*, ed. Angus Gowland (Dublin: Penguin Classics, 2021).

11 **The Hierarchical Taxonomy:** Roman Kotov et al., "The Hierarchical Taxonomy of Psychopathology (HiTOP): A Dimensional Alternative to Traditional Nosologies," *Journal of Abnormal Psychology* 126, no. 4 (May 2017): 454–77, https://doi.org/10.1037/abn0000258; Camilo J. Ruggero et al., "Integrating the Hierarchical Taxonomy of Psychopathology (HiTOP) into Clinical Practice," *Journal of Consulting and Clinical Psychology* 87, no. 12 (December 2019): 1069–84, https://doi.org/10.1037/ccp0000452.

11 Essentially, the lowest level of: Monika A. Waszczuk et al., "Redefining Phenotypes to Advance Psychiatric Genetics: Implications from Hierarchical Taxonomy of Psychopathology," *Journal of Abnormal Psychology* 129, no. 2 (February 2020): 143–61, https://doi.org/10.1037/abn0000486.

11 Research suggests that in addition: Waszczuk et al., "Redefining Phenotypes to Advance Psychiatric Genetics."

12 Studies from 2020 and 2021: Uriel Abulof, Shirley Le Penne, and Bonan Pu, "The Pandemic Politics of Existential Anxiety: Between Steadfast Resistance and Flexible Resilience," *International Political Science Review* 42, no. 3 (June 14, 2021): 350–66, https://doi.org/10.1177/01925121211002098; Noah F. G. Evers, Patricia M. Greenfield, and Gabriel W. Evers, "COVID-19 Shifts Mortality Salience, Activities, and Values in the United States: Big Data Analysis of Online Adaptation," *Human Behavior and Emerging Technologies* 3, no. 1 (January 9, 2021): 107–26, https://doi.org/10.1002/hbe2.251.

12 As recently as 2020: Alison Abbott, "COVID's Mental-Health Toll: How Scientists Are Tracking a Surge in Depression," *Nature* 590, no. 7845 (February 11, 2021): 194–95, https://doi.org/10.1038/d41586-021-00175-z; Mark É. Czeisler et al., "Mental Health, Substance Use, and Suicidal Ideation During the COVID-19 Pandemic—United States, June 24–30, 2020," *Morbidity and Mortality Weekly Report* 69, no. 32 (August 14, 2020): 1049–57, https://doi.org/10.15585/mmwr.mm6932a1.

13 In *Anxiety: A Short History*: Allan V. Horwitz, *Anxiety: A Short History* (Baltimore: Johns Hopkins University Press, 2013), 28.

13 Herbal remedies were at times prescribed: Burton, *The Anatomy of Melancholy,* 626.

14 the broad term "nervous disorders": Horwitz, *Anxiety*, 48.

14 Treatment for anxiety: Horwitz, *Anxiety*.

14 continued to emphasize: Horwitz, *Anxiety*, 53.

14 "Treatment should promote": Stanley Rachman, "The Evolution of Behaviour Therapy and Cognitive Behaviour Therapy," *Behaviour Research and Therapy* 64 (January 2015): 1–8, https://doi.org/10.1016/j.brat.2014.10.006.

15 In the 1950s: Andrea Tone, "Listening to the Past: History, Psychiatry, and Anxiety," *Canadian Journal of Psychiatry* 50, no. 7 (June 1, 2005): 373–80, https://doi.org/10.1177/070674370505000702.

16 Estimates from the: "Anxiety Disorders," World Health Organization, September 27, 2023, https://www.who.int/news-room/fact-sheets/detail/anxiety-disorders.

17 As it turns out, neuroscience: Martina de Witte et al., "Effects of Music Interventions on Stress-Related Outcomes: A Systematic Review and Two Meta-Analyses," *Health Psychology Review* 14, no. 2 (April 2, 2020): 294–324, https://doi.org/10.1080/17437199.2019.1627897.

22 Research suggests that nearly half: Ned H. Kalin, "The Critical Relationship Between Anxiety and Depression," *American Journal of Psychiatry* 177, no. 5 (May 1, 2020): 365–67, https://doi.org/10.1176/appi.ajp.2020.20030305.

23 But nothing just disappears: Sigmund Freud, *Further Remarks on the Neuro-Psychoses of Defence. Standard Edition of the Complete Psychological Works of Sigmund Freud*, vol. 3, eds. James Strachey, Anna Freud, and Anna Richards (London: Hogarth Press: 1968).

25 This plays out quite literally: Tyra Dark et al., "Epidemiology of Emergency Department Visits for Anxiety in the United States: 2009–2011," *Psychiatric Services* 68, no. 3 (March 2017): 238–44, https://doi.org/10.1176/appi.ps.201600148.

28 a growing body of evidence: Alessio Barsaglini et al., "The Effects of Psychotherapy on Brain Function: A Systematic and Critical Review," *Progress in Neurobiology* 114 (March 2014): 1–14, https://doi.org/10.1016/j.pneurobio.2013.10.006; Britta K. Hölzel et al., "Investigation of Mindfulness Meditation Practitioners with Voxel-Based Morphometry," *Social Cognitive and Affective Neuroscience* 3, no. 1 (March 1, 2008): 55–61, https://doi.org/10.1093/scan/nsm038; Benno Bremer et al., "Mindfulness Meditation Increases Default Mode, Salience, and Central Executive Network Connectivity," *Scientific Reports* 12, no. 1 (August 2, 2022): 13219, https://doi.org/10.1038/s41598-022-17325-6.

28 And research is unpacking: Steven M. Southwick and Dennis S. Charney, *Resilience: The Science of Mastering Life's Greatest Challenges* (Cambridge: Cambridge University Press, 2018).

28 In the words of: Sharon Salzberg, "Some Things Just Hurt," On Being, March 13, 2016.

29 In Roman mythology: For one of my favorite reflections on the mythology of Janus, see Jhumpa Lahiri's beautiful memoir about moving to Italy to learn Italian, *In Other Words* (New York: Knopf, 2016), in which she describes the importance of the Janus gates of Rome.

29 "Some say that": Robert Graves, *The Greek Myths*, vol. 1 (London: Penguin Books, 1960), 41.

Chapter 1: Attention

33 in sixteenth-century Italy: Luiz Severo Bem Junior et al., "The Anatomy of the Brain—Learned over the Centuries," *Surgical Neurology International* 12 (June 28, 2021): 319, https://doi.org/10.25259/SNI_200_2021; J. H. Scatliff and S. Johnston, "Andreas Vesalius and Thomas Willis: Their Anatomic Brain Illustrations and Illustrators," *American Journal of Neuroradiology* 35, no. 1 (January 2014): 19–22, https://doi.org/10.3174/ajnr.A3766.

33 in the seventeenth century: Allan V. Horwitz, *Anxiety: A Short History* (Baltimore: Johns Hopkins University Press, 2013).

36 In particular, they found lower: Jie Xu et al., "Anxious Brain Networks: A Coordinate-Based Activation Likelihood Estimation Meta-Analysis of Resting-State Functional Connectivity Studies in Anxiety," *Neuroscience & Biobehavioral Reviews* 96 (January 2019): 21–30, https://doi.org/10.1016/j.neubiorev.2018.11.005.

36 the brain has often been compared: For an extensive discussion of the comparison between the human brain and computers, see Matthew Cobb's fascinating *The Idea of the Brain: The Past and Future of Neuroscience* (New York: Basic Books, 2020).

37 Anxiety forces us to remember: The late Jeremy Safran, PhD, wrote about the ways in which we are, on a societal level, being drawn toward quick fixes: "I also believe that the current marginalization of psychoanalysis is partially attributable to certain contemporary cultural biases, especially in the United States, that are not unequivocally healthy ones. These biases include an emphasis on optimism, speed, pragmatism, instrumentality, and an intolerance of ambiguity. Although all of these emphases certainly have their value, they can also be associated with a naivete that tends to underestimate the complexity of human nature and the difficulty of the change process," *Psychoanalysis and Psychoanalytic Therapies* (Washington, DC: American Psychological Association, 2012), 7.

37 They hope to be able to: Leonardo Tozzi et al., "The Human Connectome Project for Disordered Emotional States: Protocol and Rationale for a Research Domain Criteria Study of Brain Connectivity in Young Adult Anxiety and Depression," *NeuroImage* 214 (July 2020): 116715, https://doi.org/10.1016/j.neuroimage.2020.116715.

37 looking at healthy individuals' brains: Zhihao Wang et al., "Connectome-Based Predictive Modeling of Individual Anxiety," *Cerebral Cortex* 31, no. 6 (May 10, 2021): 3006–20, https://doi.org/10.1093/cercor/bhaa407.

39 Though researchers found a: Alice V. Chavanne and Oliver J. Robinson, "The Overlapping Neurobiology of Induced and Pathological Anxiety: A Meta-Analysis of Functional Neural Activation," *American Journal of Psychiatry* 178, no. 2 (February 1, 2021): 156–64, https://doi.org/10.1176/appi.ajp.2020.19111153.

40 In the field of visual: Arien Mack and Irvin Rock, *Inattentional Blindness* (Cambridge, MA: MIT Press, 1998).

42 The World Health Organization reports: "Mental Health at Work," World Health Organization, 2024, https://www.who.int/teams/mental-health-and-substance-use/promotion-prevention/mental-health-in-the-workplace.me.

43 A seminal meta-analysis: Yair Bar-Haim et al., "Threat-Related Attentional Bias in Anxious and Nonanxious Individuals: A Meta-Analytic Study," *Psychological Bulletin* 133, no. 1 (2007): 1–24, https://doi.org/10.1037/0033-2909.133.1.1.

44 Another meta-analysis found: Catarina Botelho et al., "Neuronal Underpinnings of the Attentional Bias Toward Threat in the Anxiety Spectrum: Meta-Analytical Data on P3 and LPP Event-Related Potentials," *Biological Psychology* 176 (January 2023): 108475, https://doi.org/10.1016/j.biopsycho.2022.108475.

45 The BNST may: Lindsay K. Knight and Brendan E. Depue, "New Frontiers in Anxiety Research: The Translational Potential of the Bed Nucleus

of the Stria Terminalis," *Frontiers in Psychiatry* 10 (July 17, 2019): https://doi
.org/10.3389/fpsyt.2019.00510.

46 for people with GAD: Elena Makovac et al., "Neurostructural Abnor-
malities Associated with Axes of Emotion Dysregulation in Generalized
Anxiety," *NeuroImage: Clinical* 10 (2016): 172–81, https://doi.org/10.1016
/j.nicl.2015.11.022.

46 Researchers found that among parents: Evin Aktar et al., "Intergenerational Transmission of Attentional Bias and Anxiety," *Developmental Science* 22, no. 3 (May 13, 2019): 16, https://doi.org/10.1111/desc.12772.

47 In keeping with Shackman's description: e.g., Yafei Tan et al., "Interoceptive Attention Facilitates Emotion Regulation Strategy Use," *International Journal of Clinical and Health Psychology* 23, no. 1 (January 2023):
100336, https://doi.org/10.1016/j.ijchp.2022.100336; Julian F. Thayer and
Richard D. Lane, "A Model of Neurovisceral Integration in Emotion Regulation and Dysregulation," *Journal of Affective Disorders* 61, no. 3 (December 2000): 201–16, https://doi.org/10.1016/S0165-0327(00)00338-4; Heather
A. Wadlinger and Derek M. Isaacowitz. "Fixing Our Focus: Training Attention to Regulate Emotion," *Personality and Social Psychology Review* 15,
no. 1 (February 2011): 75–102, https://doi.org/10.1177/1088868310365565.

47 having a degree of control: Joseph R. Bardeen et al., "Attentional Control
as a Moderator of the Relationship Between Difficulties Accessing Effective Emotion Regulation Strategies and Distress Tolerance," *Journal of
Psychopathology and Behavioral Assessment* 37, no. 1 (March 17, 2015): 79–84,
https://doi.org/10.1007/s10862-014-9433-2.

49 In the now classic book: Jonathan Kabat-Zinn, *Full Catastrophe Living:
Using the Wisdom of Your Body and Mind to Face Stress, Pain, and Illness*
(New York: Bantam Books, 2013), 21.

49 And though MBSR: Jon Kabat-Zinn, "Some Reflections on the Origins
of MBSR, Skillful Means, and the Trouble with Maps," *Contemporary
Buddhism* 12, no. 1 (May 1, 2011): 281–306, https://doi.org/10.1080/14639947
.2011.564844.

50 MBSR has been found: E.g., Daniel C. Cherkin et al., "Effect of
Mindfulness-Based Stress Reduction vs. Cognitive Behavioral Therapy or
Usual Care on Back Pain and Functional Limitations in Adults with Chronic

Low Back Pain," *JAMA* 315, no. 12 (March 22, 2016): 1240, https://doi.org/10.1001/jama.2016.2323; Ciro Conversano et al., "Is Mindfulness-Based Stress Reduction Effective for People with Hypertension? A Systematic Review and Meta-Analysis of 30 Years of Evidence," *International Journal of Environmental Research and Public Health* 18, no. 6 (March 11, 2021): 2882, https://doi.org/10.3390/ijerph18062882; Estelle T. Higgins et al., "Clinically Relevant Effects of Mindfulness-Based Stress Reduction in Individuals with Asthma," *Brain, Behavior, & Immunity—Health* 25 (November 2022): 100509, https://doi.org/10.1016/j.bbih.2022.100509.

50 **a reduction in symptoms:** E.g., Jon Vøllestad, Børge Sivertsen, and Geir Høstmark Nielsen, "Mindfulness-Based Stress Reduction for Patients with Anxiety Disorders: Evaluation in a Randomized Controlled Trial," *Behaviour Research and Therapy* 49, no. 4 (April 2011): 281–88, https://doi.org/10.1016/j.brat.2011.01.007.

50 **MBSR was as effective:** Elizabeth A. Hoge et al., "Mindfulness-Based Stress Reduction vs. Escitalopram for the Treatment of Adults with Anxiety Disorders," *JAMA Psychiatry* 80, no. 1 (January 1, 2023): 13, https://doi.org/10.1001/jamapsychiatry.2022.3679.

51 **Barbara Oakley, PhD, an engineer:** Barbara Oakley, *A Mind for Numbers: How to Excel at Math and Science* (New York: TarcherPerigee, 2014), 11.

52 **More recently, flow has been:** Julia Zielke, Manuel Anglada-Tort, and Jonathan Berger, "Inducing and Disrupting Flow During Music Performance," *Frontiers in Psychology* 14 (June 2, 2023): 1, https://doi.org/10.3389/fpsyg.2023.1187153.

53 **Flow can even be:** Amy Rakei, Jasmine Tan, and Joydeep Bhattacharya, "Flow in Contemporary Musicians: Individual Differences in Flow Proneness, Anxiety, and Emotional Intelligence," *PLOS ONE* 17, no. 3 (March 25, 2022): e0265936, https://doi.org/10.1371/journal.pone.0265936.

53 **only through tolerating the discomfort:** Josh Dickson, "Using Flow Science to Help Your Clients Thrive," Presentation at The Master Series, Oxford, England, September 1, 2023.

53 **A truly ancient art form:** Kassia St. Clair, *The Golden Thread: How Fabric Changed History* (New York: Liveright Publishing Corporation, 2019).

53 I later learned that sashiko: Susan Briscoe, *The Ultimate Sashiko Sourcebook* (Exeter, UK: David and Charles, Ltd., 2004), 8.

54 found only negligible differences: Anita Harrewijn et al., "Cortical and Subcortical Brain Structure in Generalized Anxiety Disorder: Findings from 28 Research Sites in the ENIGMA-Anxiety Working Group," *Translational Psychiatry* 11, no. 1 (December 1, 2021): 502, https://doi.org/10.1038/s41398-021-01622-1.

54 But despite so much promise: Scott Marek et al., "Reproducible Brain-Wide Association Studies Require Thousands of Individuals," *Nature* 603, no. 7902 (March 24, 2022): 654–60, https://doi.org/10.1038/s41586-022-04492-9.

Chapter 2: Curiosity and Flexibility

57 Why is it: Researchers who study the impact of psychedelics on mental health describe "stuck states" saying, "mental illness or psychopathology is the result of being confined to a rigid, single state (stuck state), unable to transition between states, leading to maladaptive thoughts, emotions, and behaviours." Inês Hipólito et al., "Pattern Breaking: A Complex Systems Approach to Psychedelic Medicine," *Neuroscience of Consciousness* 2023, no. 1 (July 6, 2023): 7, https://doi.org/10.1093/nc/niad017.

57 As the oft-quoted saying: Carla J. Shatz, "The Developing Brain," *Scientific American* 267, no. 3 (September 1992): 60–67, https://doi.org/10.1038/scientificamerican0992-60; Donald Hebb, *The Organization of Behavior* (New York: John Wiley and Sons, 1949).

58 The CSTC loop: Wayne K. Goodman, Eric A. Storch, and Sameer A. Sheth, "Harmonizing the Neurobiology and Treatment of Obsessive-Compulsive Disorder," *American Journal of Psychiatry* 178, no. 1 (January 1, 2021): 17–29, https://doi.org/10.1176/appi.ajp.2020.20111601.

58 OCD is defined: Roseli G. Shavitt et al., "Phenomenology of OCD: Lessons from a Large Multicenter Study and Implications for ICD-11," *Journal of Psychiatric Research* 57 (October 2014): 141–48, https://doi.org/10.1016/j.jpsychires.2014.06.010; *Diagnostic and Statistical Manual of Mental Disorders* (Washington, DC: American Psychiatric Association, 2013).

60 in a sample of fifteen thousand: Eesha Sharma et al., "Comorbidities in Obsessive-Compulsive Disorder Across the Lifespan: A Systematic Review and Meta-Analysis," *Frontiers in Psychiatry* 12 (November 11, 2021): https://doi.org/10.3389/fpsyt.2021.703701.

61 Abramowitz, along with psychologist Ryan Jacoby: Jonathan S. Abramowitz and Ryan J. Jacoby, "Obsessive-Compulsive Disorder in the DSM-5," *Clinical Psychology: Science and Practice* 21, no. 3 (September 2014): 221–35, https://doi.org/10.1111/cpsp.12076; Jonathan S. Abramowitz and Ryan J. Jacoby, "Obsessive-Compulsive and Related Disorders: A Critical Review of the New Diagnostic Class," *Annual Review of Clinical Psychology* 11, no. 1 (March 28, 2015): 165–86, https://doi.org/10.1146/annurev-clinpsy-032813-153713.

61 Applied to obsessions: E.g., Stanley Rachman and Ray Hodgson, *Obsessions and Compulsions* (Englewood Cliffs, NJ: Prentice-Hall, 1980).

61 Rachman refers to: Rachman and Hodgson, *Obsessions and Compulsions*, 252.

63 the five components: Lauren S. Hallion et al., "A Five-Factor Model of Perseverative Thought," *Journal of Psychopathology and Clinical Science* (February 7, 2022): 16, https://doi.org/10.1037/abn0000737.

64 anxiety is associated with: Junchol Park and Bita Moghaddam, "Impact of Anxiety on Prefrontal Cortex Encoding of Cognitive Flexibility," *Neuroscience* 345 (March 2017): 193–202, https://doi.org/10.1016/j.neuroscience.2016.06.013.

64 people with GAD and OCD: Ángel Rosa-Alcázar et al., "Cognitive Flexibility and Response Inhibition in Patients with Obsessive-Compulsive Disorder and Generalized Anxiety Disorder," *International Journal of Clinical and Health Psychology* 20, no. 1 (January 2020): 20–28, https://doi.org/10.1016/j.ijchp.2019.07.006.

65 emotional rigidity got: Anika Wiltgen et al., "Emotional Rigidity Negatively Impacts Remission from Anxiety and Recovery of Well-Being," *Journal of Affective Disorders* 236 (August 2018): 69–74, https://doi.org/10.1016/j.jad.2018.04.113.

65 "the processes by which": James J. Gross, "The Emerging Field of Emotion Regulation: An Integrative Review," *Review of General Psychology* 2, no. 3 (September 1, 1998): 271–99, 275, https://doi.org/10.1037/1089-2680

.2.3.271; James J. Gross, "Emotion Regulation: Current Status and Future Prospects," *Psychological Inquiry* 26, no. 1 (January 2, 2015): 1–26, https://doi.org/10.1080/1047840X.2014.940781; Allison S. Troy et al., "Psychological Resilience: An Affect-Regulation Framework," *Annual Review of Psychology* 74, no. 1 (January 18, 2023): 547–76, https://doi.org/10.1146/annurev-psych-020122-041854.

65 **lower levels of resilience:** Joseph M Diehl, "Emotion Regulation Difficulties Link Trait Resilience and Symptoms of Depression and Anxiety in Psychiatric Outpatients," *Annals of Clinical Psychiatry* 34, no. 4 (November 2022): https://doi.org/10.12788/acp.0086.

66 **higher levels of impulsivity:** E.g., Alessandra Del Carlo et al., "Different Measures of Impulsivity in Patients with Anxiety Disorders: A Case Control Study," *Psychiatry Research* 197, no. 3 (May 2012): 231–36, https://doi.org/10.1016/j.psychres.2011.09.020.

68 **Stuart Vyse, a psychologist:** Stuart Vyse, *Believing in Magic: The Psychology of Superstition* (Oxford: Oxford University Press, 2014), 243.

72 **Most of all, Becker writes:** Ernest Becker, *The Denial of Death* (New York: Free Press, 1973), xvii.

72 **In the 1980s, Becker's work:** Sheldon Solomon, Jeff Greenberg, and Tom Pyszczynski, *The Worm at the Core: On the Role of Death in Life* (New York: Random House, 2015).

72 **According to TMT:** E.g., Jeff Greenberg et al., "Why Do People Need Self-Esteem? Converging Evidence That Self-Esteem Serves an Anxiety-Buffering Function," *Journal of Personality and Social Psychology* 63, no. 6 (1992): 913–22, https://doi.org/10.1037/0022-3514.63.6.913.

72 **With this buffer in place:** Greenberg et al., "Why Do People Need Self-Esteem?"

73 **among people with OCD:** E.g., Rachel E. Verin, Rachel E. Menzies, and Ross G. Menzies, "OCD, Death Anxiety, and Attachment: What's Love Got to Do with It?," *Behavioural and Cognitive Psychotherapy* 50, no. 2 (March 2, 2022): 131–41, https://doi.org/10.1017/S135246582100045X; Rachel E. Menzies and Ilan Dar-Nimrod, "Death Anxiety and Its Relationship with Obsessive-Compulsive Disorder," *Journal of Abnormal Psychology* 126, no. 4 (May 2017): 367–77, https://doi.org/10.1037/abn0000263.

73 These participants literally used: Menzies and Dar-Nimrod, "Death Anxiety and Its Relationship with Obsessive-Compulsive Disorder."

74 the term "anankastia": *International Classification of Diseases, Eleventh Revision (ICD-11)*, 11th ed. (Geneva: World Health Organization, 2022), https://icd.who.int/.

74 Robert Burton described: Robert Burton, *The Anatomy of Melancholy*, ed. Angus Gowland (Dublin: Penguin Classics, 2021), 377.

75 when negative emotions: David H. Rosmarin and Bethany Leidl, "Spirituality, Religion, and Anxiety Disorders," *Handbook of Spirituality, Religion, and Mental Health*, 2020: 41–60, https://doi.org/10.1016/B978-0-12-816766 -3.00003-3.

76 Yale-Brown Obsessive-Compulsive Scale: Wayne K. Goodman et al., "The Yale-Brown Obsessive Compulsive Scale: I. Development, Use, and Reliability," *Archives of General Psychiatry* 46, no. 11 (November 1, 1989): 1006, https://doi.org/10.1001/archpsyc.1989.01810110048007.

77 ERP, widely considered: E.g., V. Nezgovorova et al., "Optimizing First Line Treatments for Adults with OCD," *Comprehensive Psychiatry* 115 (May 2022): 152305, https://doi.org/10.1016/j.comppsych.2022.152305.

78 Though research in this area: E.g., Kristoffer A. A. Andersen et al., "Therapeutic Effects of Classic Serotonergic Psychedelics: A Systematic Review of Modern-Era Clinical Studies," *Acta Psychiatrica Scandinavica* 143, no. 2 (February 2021): 101–18, https://doi.org/10.1111/acps.13249; Iman Khan et al., "Use of Selective Alternative Therapies for Treatment of OCD," *Neuropsychiatric Disease and Treatment* Volume 19 (April 2023): 721–32, https://doi.org/10.2147/NDT.S403997; Silvia Muttoni, Maddalena Ardissino, and Christopher John, "Classical Psychedelics for the Treatment of Depression and Anxiety: A Systematic Review," *Journal of Affective Disorders* 258 (November 2019): 11–24, https://doi.org/10.1016/j.jad.2019 .07.076.

78 In a recent paper: Hipólito et al., "Pattern Breaking," 1.

79 "Carefulness, the application": "Curiosity, n.," OED Online, Oxford University Press, 2022, https://www.oed.com/dictionary/curiosity_n?tl =true.

79 Daniel Siegel, a psychiatrist: "Daniel Siegel: Name It to Tame It," Daniel Siegel, Dalai Lama Center for Peace and Education, YouTube, December 8, 2014, https://www.youtube.com/watch?v=ZcDLzppD4Jc.

79 Research on affect labeling: Matthew D. Lieberman et al., "Subjective Responses to Emotional Stimuli during Labeling, Reappraisal, and Distraction," *Emotion* 11, no. 3 (June 2011): 468–80, https://doi.org/10.1037/a0023503; Lisa Feldman Barrett, *How Emotions Are Made: The Secret Life of the Brain* (New York: Houghton Mifflin Harcourt Publishing Company, 2017).

Chapter 3: Boundaries and Permeability

87 In the classic: Henry Gray, *Gray's Anatomy*, ed. T. Pickering Pick and Robert Howden (New York: Running Press, 1974), 1077.

87 Humoral theory integrated: Roy Porter, *The Greatest Benefit to Mankind: A Medical History of Humanity* (New York: W. W. Norton & Company, Inc, 1997), 9.

88 a strong genetic component: E.g., Mihoko Shimada-Sugimoto, Takeshi Otowa, and John M. Hettema, "Genetics of Anxiety Disorders: Genetic Epidemiological and Molecular Studies in Humans," *Psychiatry and Clinical Neurosciences* 69, no. 7 (July 5, 2015): 388–401, https://doi.org/10.1111/pcn.12291.

89 We know that: M. A. Schiele and K. Domschke, "Epigenetics at the Crossroads between Genes, Environment and Resilience in Anxiety Disorders," *Genes, Brain and Behavior* 17, no. 3 (March 2018): e12423, 2, https://doi.org/10.1111/gbb.12423.

89 Twin studies on: E.g., John M. Hettema et al., "The Structure of Genetic and Environmental Risk Factors for Anxiety Disorders in Men and Women," *Archives of General Psychiatry* 62, no. 2 (February 1, 2005): 182, https://doi.org/10.1001/archpsyc.62.2.182.

89 Genome-wide association studies: E.g., Maija-Kreetta Koskinen and Iiris Hovatta, "Genetic Insights into the Neurobiology of Anxiety," *Trends in Neurosciences* 46, no. 4 (April 2023): 318–31, https://doi.org/10.1016/j.tins.2023.01.007.

90 **our genetics and our experiences:** Rujia Wang, Catharina A. Hartman, and Harold Snieder, "Stress-Related Exposures Amplify the Effects of Genetic Susceptibility on Depression and Anxiety," *Translational Psychiatry* 13, no. 1 (January 30, 2023): 27, https://doi.org/10.1038/s41398-023-02327-3.

90 **think about the inheritance:** Helga Ask et al., "Genetic Contributions to Anxiety Disorders: Where We Are and Where We Are Heading," *Psychological Medicine* 51, no. 13 (October 9, 2021): 2231–46, https://doi.org/10.1017/S0033291720005486.

90 **genetics of anxiety disorders:** Daniel F. Levey et al., "Reproducible Genetic Risk Loci for Anxiety: Results From ~200,000 Participants in the Million Veteran Program," *American Journal of Psychiatry* 177, no. 3 (March 1, 2020): 223–32, https://doi.org/10.1176/appi.ajp.2019.19030256; Kazutaka Ohi et al., "Shared Genetic Etiology Between Anxiety Disorders and Psychiatric and Related Intermediate Phenotypes," *Psychological Medicine* 50, no. 4 (March 28, 2020): 692–704, https://doi.org/10.1017/S003329171900059X.

91 **compared using genomically assisted:** John Papastergiou et al., "Pharmacogenomics Guided versus Standard Antidepressant Treatment in a Community Pharmacy Setting: A Randomized Controlled Trial," *Clinical and Translational Science* 14, no. 4 (July 28, 2021): 1359–68, https://doi.org/10.1111/cts.12986.

91 **But much remains:** Ahmed Z. Elmaadawi et al., "Effect of Pharmacogenomic Testing on Pediatric Mental Health Outcome: A 6-Month Follow-Up," *Pharmacogenomics* 24, no. 2 (January 2023): 73–82, https://doi.org/10.2217/pgs-2022-0131.

92 **a number of factors:** Catherine R. Virelli, Ayeshah G. Mohiuddin, and James L. Kennedy, "Barriers to Clinical Adoption of Pharmacogenomic Testing in Psychiatry: A Critical Analysis," *Translational Psychiatry* 11, no. 1 (December 6, 2021): 509, https://doi.org/10.1038/s41398-021-01600-7.

97 **Sometimes, changes in the blood:** Anthony W. Austin, Stephen M. Patterson, and Roland von Känel, "Hemoconcentration and Hemostasis During Acute Stress: Interacting and Independent Effects," *Annals of Behavioral Medicine* 42, no. 2 (October 12, 2011): 153–73, https://doi.org/10.1007/s12160-011-9274-0; Anthony Austin, Thomas Wissmann, and Roland von Kanel, "Stress and Hemostasis: An Update," *Seminars in*

Thrombosis and Hemostasis 39, no. 8 (October 10, 2013): 902–12, https://doi.org/10.1055/s-0033-1357487.

97 **Acute stress can:** Roland von Känel, "Acute Mental Stress and Hemostasis: When Physiology Becomes Vascular Harm," *Thrombosis Research* 135 (February 2015): S52–55, https://doi.org/10.1016/S0049-3848(15)50444-1; Roland Von Känel et al., "Effects of Psychological Stress and Psychiatric Disorders on Blood Coagulation and Fibrinolysis: A Biobehavioral Pathway to Coronary Artery Disease?," *Psychosomatic Medicine* 63, no. 4 (July 2001): 531–44, https://doi.org/10.1097/00006842-200107000-00003.

98 **increases in inflammatory:** Ruihua Hou et al., "Peripheral Inflammatory Cytokines and Immune Balance in Generalised Anxiety Disorder: Case-Controlled Study," *Brain, Behavior, and Immunity* 62 (May 2017): 212–18, https://doi.org/10.1016/j.bbi.2017.01.021; Zhen Tang et al., "Peripheral Proinflammatory Cytokines in Chinese Patients with Generalised Anxiety Disorder," *Journal of Affective Disorders* 225 (January 2018): 593–98, https://doi.org/10.1016/j.jad.2017.08.082; Christiaan H. Vinkers et al., "An Integrated Approach to Understand Biological Stress System Dysregulation across Depressive and Anxiety Disorders," *Journal of Affective Disorders* 283 (March 2021): 139–46, https://doi.org/10.1016/j.jad.2021.01.051.

99 **increased pro-inflammatory cytokines:** Megan E. Renna et al., "The Association Between Anxiety, Traumatic Stress, and Obsessive-Compulsive Disorders and Chronic Inflammation: A Systematic Review and Meta-Analysis," *Depression and Anxiety* 35, no. 11 (November 2018): 1081–94, https://doi.org/10.1002/da.22790.

99 **generalized anxiety disorder and inflammation:** Harry Costello et al., "Systematic Review and Meta-Analysis of the Association Between Peripheral Inflammatory Cytokines and Generalised Anxiety Disorder," *British Medical Journal Open* 9, no. 7 (July 19, 2019): e027925, https://doi.org/10.1136/bmjopen-2018-027925.

99 **Remarkably, there is:** Piotr Gałecki, Joanna Mossakowska-Wójcik, and Monika Talarowska, "The Anti-Inflammatory Mechanism of Antidepressants—SSRIs, SNRIs," *Progress in Neuro-Psychopharmacology and Biological Psychiatry* 80 (January 2018): 291–94, https://doi.org/10.1016/j.pnpbp.2017.03.016; Ruihua Hou et al., "Effects of SSRIs on Peripheral Inflammatory Cytokines in Patients with Generalized Anxiety Disorder,"

Brain, Behavior, and Immunity 81 (October 2019): 105–10, https://doi.org/10.1016 /j.bbi.2019.06.001; Yukitoshi Izumi et al., "SSRIs Differentially Modulate the Effects of Pro-Inflammatory Stimulation on Hippocampal Plasticity and Memory via Sigma 1 Receptors and Neurosteroids," *Translational Psychiatry* 13, no. 1 (February 3, 2023): 39, https://doi.org/10.1038/s41398-023-02343-3; Shrujna Patel, Brooke A. Keating, and Russell C. Dale, "Anti-Inflammatory Properties of Commonly Used Psychiatric Drugs," *Frontiers in Neuroscience* 16 (January 10, 2023): https://doi.org/10.3389/fnins.2022.1039379.

99 **ways that techniques:** E.g., Erin M. Ellis et al., "Direct and Indirect Associations of Cognitive Reappraisal and Suppression with Disease Biomarkers," *Psychology & Health* 34, no. 3 (March 4, 2019): 336–54, https:// doi.org/10.1080/08870446.2018.1529313.

100 **Psychologist Megan Renna:** Megan E. Renna, "A Review and Novel Theoretical Model of How Negative Emotions Influence Inflammation: The Critical Role of Emotion Regulation," *Brain, Behavior, & Immunity—Health* 18 (December 2021): 100397, https://doi.org/10.1016/j.bbih.2021.100397.

100 **A burgeoning scar model:** Nur Hani Zainal and Michelle G. Newman, "Elevated Anxious and Depressed Mood Relates to Future Executive Dysfunction in Older Adults: A Longitudinal Network Analysis of Psychopathology and Cognitive Functioning," *Clinical Psychological Science* 11, no. 2 (March 14, 2023): 218–38, https://doi.org/10.1177/21677026221114076.

101 **Higher levels of anxiety:** Nur Hani Zainal and Michelle G. Newman, "Depression and Worry Symptoms Predict Future Executive Functioning Impairment via Inflammation," *Psychological Medicine* 52, no. 15 (November 3, 2022): 3625–35, https://doi.org/10.1017/S0033291721000398.

101 **Again, they found that depression:** Nur Hani Zainal and Michelle G. Newman, "Inflammation Mediates Depression and Generalized Anxiety Symptoms Predicting Executive Function Impairment after 18 Years," *Journal of Affective Disorders* 296 (January 2022): 465–75, https://doi.org /10.1016/j.jad.2021.08.077.

Chapter 4: A Force to Be Reckoned With

106 **History shows us:** John Meletis and Kostas Konstantopoulos, "The Beliefs, Myths, and Reality Surrounding the Word Hema (Blood) from Homer to the Present," *Anemia* 2010 (2010): 1–6, https://doi.org/10.1155/2010/857657.

106 **"Pliny recorded epileptics":** Nick Groom, *The Vampire: A New History* (New Haven, CT: Yale University Press, 2018), 10–11.

106 **Dragon's blood has:** Deepika Gupta, Bruce Bleakley, and Rajinder K. Gupta, "Dragon's Blood: Botany, Chemistry and Therapeutic Uses," *Journal of Ethnopharmacology* 115, no. 3 (February 2008): 361–80, https://doi .org/10.1016/j.jep.2007.10.018; Victoria Pickering, "Plant of the Month: The Dragon Tree," JSTOR Daily, July 1, 2020.

106 **And in laboratory:** Gupta, Bleakley, and Gupta, "Dragon's Blood: Botany, Chemistry and Therapeutic Uses."

107 **William Harvey, an English physician:** Domenico Ribatti, "William Harvey and the Discovery of the Circulation of the Blood," *Journal of Angiogenesis Research* 1, no. 1 (2009): 3, https://doi.org/10.1186/2040-2384-1-3.

107 **"It is absolutely necessary":** William Harvey, *On the Motion of the Heart and Blood in Animals: A New Edition of William Harvey's Exercitatio Anatomica de Motu Cordis et Sanguinis in Animalibus*, ed. Jarrett A. Carty (Eugene, OR: Resource Publications, 2016), 76.

109 **This bears out in data:** E.g., R. Nicholas Carleton, "Into the Unknown: A Review and Synthesis of Contemporary Models Involving Uncertainty," *Journal of Anxiety Disorders* 39 (April 2016): 30–43, https://doi.org/10.1016 /j.janxdis.2016.02.007.

109 **"Yet their bodies are":** Robert Burton, *The Anatomy of Melancholy*, ed. Angus Gowland (Dublin: Penguin Classics, 2021), 380.

109 **The current (much drier):** *Diagnostic and Statistical Manual of Mental Disorders* (Washington, DC: American Psychiatric Association, 2013), 315.

111 **The term "safety behavior":** E.g., S. Rachman, "Agoraphobia—A Safety-Signal Perspective," *Behaviour Research and Therapy* 22, no. 1 (1984): 59–70, https://doi.org/10.1016/0005-7967(84)90033-0; Paul M. Salkovskis, "The Importance of Behaviour in the Maintenance of Anxiety and Panic: A Cognitive Account," *Behavioural Psychotherapy* 19, no. 1 (January 16, 1991): 6–19, https://doi.org/10.1017/S0141347300011472.

112 **although safety behaviors:** Sylvia Helbig-Lang and Franz Petermann, "Tolerate or Eliminate? A Systematic Review on the Effects of Safety Behavior across Anxiety Disorders," *Clinical Psychology: Science and Practice*

17, no. 3 (September 2010): 218–33, https://doi.org/10.1111/j.1468-2850.2010 .01213.x.

112 **In 1994, in a now classic paper:** S. Woody and S. Rachman, "Generalized Anxiety Disorder (GAD) as an Unsuccessful Search for Safety," *Clinical Psychology Review* 14, no. 8 (January 1994): 743–53, 750, https://doi.org /10.1016/0272-7358(94)90040-X.

112 **The term "cyberchondria":** Vladan Starcevic, David Berle, and Sandra Arnáez, "Recent Insights into Cyberchondria," *Current Psychiatry Reports* 22, no. 11 (November 27, 2020): 56, https://doi.org/10.1007/s11920-020 -01179-8.

113 **argues that cyberchondria:** Sandra K. Schenkel et al., "Conceptualizations of Cyberchondria and Relations to the Anxiety Spectrum: Systematic Review and Meta-Analysis," *Journal of Medical Internet Research* 23, no. 11 (November 18, 2021): e27835, https://doi.org/10.2196/27835.

114 **Heart disease, whose:** "Leading Causes of Death—Females—All Races and Origins—United States, 2018," Centers for Disease Control and Prevention, https://www.cdc.gov/women/lcod/2018/all-races-origins/index .htm.

114 **In *Unwell Women*:** Elinor Cleghorn, *Unwell Women: A Journey Through Medicine and Myth in a Man-Made World* (New York: Dutton, 2021), 3.

115 **the impact of structural racism:** Zinzi D. Bailey et al., "Structural Racism and Health Inequities in the USA: Evidence and Interventions," *The Lancet* 389, no. 10077 (April 2017): 1453–63, https://doi.org/10.1016/S0140 -6736(17)30569-X.

116 **with health anxiety *maintain*:** Congrong Shi et al., "Attentional Bias Toward Health-Threat in Health Anxiety: A Systematic Review and Three-Level Meta-Analysis," *Psychological Medicine* (January 10, 2022): 1–10, https://doi.org/10.1017/S0033291721005432.

116 **some people with health anxiety:** Travis A. Rogers, Thomas A. Daniel, and Joseph R. Bardeen, "Health Anxiety and Attentional Control Interact to Predict Uncertainty-Related Attentional Biases," *Journal of Behavior Therapy and Experimental Psychiatry* 74 (March 2022): 101697, https://doi .org/10.1016/j.jbtep.2021.101697.

120 It has been: Michael Hickey, "Why Is Hemophilia Called the Royal Disease?," Hemaware.org, https://hemaware.org/bleeding-disorders-z/royal -disease, April 28, 2023.

121 The word "hematopoiesis": Éva Mezey, "On the Origin of Blood Cells— Hematopoiesis Revisited," *Oral Diseases* 22, no. 4 (May 2016): 247–48, https://doi.org/10.1111/odi.12445.

122 fetal immune system: Niklas W. Andersson et al., "Influence of Prenatal Maternal Stress on Umbilical Cord Blood Cytokine Levels," *Archives of Women's Mental Health* 19, no. 5 (October 5, 2016): 761–67, https://doi.org /10.1007/s00737-016-0607-7.

122 IL-7 is known: Cédric Galera et al., "Cord Serum Cytokines at Birth and Children's Anxiety-Depression Trajectories From 3 to 8 Years: The EDEN Mother-Child Cohort," *Biological Psychiatry* 89, no. 6 (March 2021): 541–49, https://doi.org/10.1016/j.biopsych.2020.10.009.

122 Telomeres, which were: Glenn Verner et al., "Maternal Psychological Resilience During Pregnancy and Newborn Telomere Length: A Prospective Study," *American Journal of Psychiatry* 178, no. 2 (February 1, 2021): 183–92, https://doi.org/10.1176/appi.ajp.2020.19101003.

123 "the placenta provides": Hayley Dingsdale et al., "The Placenta Protects the Fetal Circulation from Anxiety-Driven Elevations in Maternal Serum Levels of Brain-Derived Neurotrophic Factor," *Translational Psychiatry* 11, no. 1 (January 18, 2021): 62, https://doi.org/10.1038/s41398-020-01176-8.

Chapter 5: Regulation and Perseverance

127 in the Hippocratic Corpus: Hippocrates, *Hippocratic Writings*, ed. G. E. R. Lloyd (London: Penguin, 1950), 250.

128 In the early seventeenth century: Robert Burton, *The Anatomy of Melancholy*, ed. Angus Gowland (Dublin: Penguin Classics, 2021), 375.

129 People in the midst: *Diagnostic and Statistical Manual of Mental Disorders* (Washington, DC: American Psychiatric Association, 2013), 208.

132 Interoception encompasses multiple: Swarna Buddha Nayok et al., "A Primer on Interoception and Its Importance in Psychiatry," *Clinical Psychopharmacology and Neuroscience* 21, no. 2 (May 30, 2023): 252–61, https://doi

.org/10.9758/cpn.2023.21.2.252; Sarah N. Garfinkel et al., "Knowing Your Own Heart: Distinguishing Interoceptive Accuracy from Interoceptive Awareness," *Biological Psychology* 104 (January 2015): 65–74, https://doi .org/10.1016/j.biopsycho.2014.11.004.

132 **In thinking through:** Kiera Louise Adams et al., "The Association Between Anxiety and Cardiac Interoceptive Accuracy: A Systematic Review and Meta-Analysis," *Neuroscience & Biobehavioral Reviews* 140 (September 2022): 104754, https://doi.org/10.1016/j.neubiorev.2022.104754.

133 **distress tolerance is defined as both:** Teresa M. Leyro, Michael J. Zvo-lensky, and Amit Bernstein, "Distress Tolerance and Psychopathological Symptoms and Disorders: A Review of the Empirical Literature among Adults," *Psychological Bulletin* 136, no. 4 (July 2010): 576–600, https://doi .org/10.1037/a0019712.

133 **Though Linehan is:** Marsha M. Linehan and Chelsey R. Wilks, "The Course and Evolution of Dialectical Behavior Therapy," *American Journal of Psychotherapy* 69, no. 2 (April 2015): 97–110, https://doi.org/10.1176/appi .psychotherapy.2015.69.2.97.

134 **People who are:** E.g., Judith M. Laposa et al., "Distress Tolerance in OCD and Anxiety Disorders, and Its Relationship with Anxiety Sensitivity and Intolerance of Uncertainty," *Journal of Anxiety Disorders* 33 (June 2015): 8–14, https://doi.org/10.1016/j.janxdis.2015.04.003.

134 **Indeed, distress tolerance:** Meghan E. Keough et al., "Anxiety Symptomatology: The Association with Distress Tolerance and Anxiety Sensitivity," *Behavior Therapy* 41, no. 4 (December 2010): 567–74, https://doi.org /10.1016/j.beth.2010.04.002.

135 **mindfulness seems to be helpful:** Yanjuan Li et al., "Distress Tolerance as a Mechanism of Mindfulness for Depression and Anxiety: Cross-Sectional and Diary Evidence," *International Journal of Clinical and Health Psychology* 23, no. 4 (October 2023): 100392, https://doi.org/10.1016/j.ijchp.2023.100392.

135 **"Each of us":** Daniel J. Siegel, *The Developing Mind: How Relationships and the Brain Interact to Shape Who We Are* (New York: Guilford Press, 2020), 341.

135 **Elizabeth Stanley, PhD, an expert:** Elizabeth A. Stanley, *Widen the Window: Training Your Brain and Body to Thrive During Stress and Recover from Trauma* (London: Yellow Kite, 2019), 104.

136 Biofeedback training is: E.g., V. C. Goessl, J. E. Curtiss, and S. G. Hofmann, "The Effect of Heart Rate Variability Biofeedback Training on Stress and Anxiety: A Meta-Analysis," *Psychological Medicine* 47, no. 15 (November 8, 2017): 2578–86, https://doi.org/10.1017/S0033291717001003; Poppy L. A. Schoenberg and Anthony S. David, "Biofeedback for Psychiatric Disorders: A Systematic Review," *Applied Psychophysiology and Biofeedback* 39, no. 2 (June 8, 2014): 109–35, https://doi.org/10.1007/s10484-014-9246-9.

137 Anxiety and obsessive-compulsive disorder: Sheharyar Minhas et al., "Mind-Body Connection: Cardiovascular Sequelae of Psychiatric Illness," *Current Problems in Cardiology* 47, no. 10 (October 2022): 100959, https://doi .org/10.1016/j.cpcardiol.2021.100959.

138 Anxiety and hypertension: Tingting Qiu et al., "Comorbidity of Anxiety and Hypertension: Common Risk Factors and Potential Mechanisms," *International Journal of Hypertension* 2023 (May 25, 2023): 1–14, https://doi .org/10.1155/2023/9619388.

138 In a large meta-analysis: Italics added. Li-Faye Lim, Marco Solmi, and Samuele Cortese, "Association Between Anxiety and Hypertension in Adults: A Systematic Review and Meta-Analysis," *Neuroscience & Biobehavioral Reviews* 131 (December 2021): 96–119, https://doi.org/10.1016/j .neubiorev.2021.08.031.

138 Another team of researchers: Chuka Mike Ifeagwazi, Helen Eleh Egberi, and JohnBosco Chika Chukwuorji, "Emotional Reactivity and Blood Pressure Elevations: Anxiety as a Mediator," *Psychology, Health & Medicine* 23, no. 5 (May 28, 2018): 585–92, https://doi.org/10.1080/13548506.2017 .1400670.

138 Healthy HRV indicates: E.g., Andre Pittig et al., "Heart Rate and Heart Rate Variability in Panic, Social Anxiety, Obsessive-Compulsive, and Generalized Anxiety Disorders at Baseline and in Response to Relaxation and Hyperventilation," *International Journal of Psychophysiology* 87, no. 1 (January 2013): 19–27, https://doi.org/10.1016/j.ijpsycho.2012.10.012.

139 The following year: Stephen W. Porges, "Orienting in a Defensive World: Mammalian Modifications of Our Evolutionary Heritage. A Polyvagal Theory," *Psychophysiology* 32, no. 4 (July 1995): 301–18, https://doi.org/10 .1111/j.1469-8986.1995.tb01213.x.

139 **Porges writes that:** Stephen W. Porges, "Polyvagal Theory: A Science of Safety," *Frontiers in Integrative Neuroscience* 16 (May 10, 2022): 1, https://doi .org/10.3389/fnint.2022.871227.

139 **With polyvagal theory:** Stephen W. Porges, "The Polyvagal Perspective," *Biological Psychology* 74, no. 2 (February 2007): 116–43, https://doi.org /10.1016/j.biopsycho.2006.06.009.

140 **Porges explains that "the polyvagal theory":** Stephen W. Porges, *The Polyvagal Theory: Neurophysiological Foundations of Emotions, Attachment, Communication, Self-Regulation* (New York: W. W. Norton & Company, 2011), 20.

140 **According to polyvagal theory:** Stephen W. Porges, *The Polyvagal Perspective.*

140 **Fundamentally, these polyvagal:** Stephen W. Porges, *The Pocket Guide to Polyvagal Theory: The Transformative Power of Feeling Safe*; Stephen W. Porges, "Polyvagal Theory: A Biobehavioral Journey to Sociality," *Comprehensive Psychoneuroendocrinology* 7 (August 2021): 100069, https://doi.org /10.1016/j.cpnec.2021.100069.

141 **Soon after speaking with him:** Stephen Porges, Bessel van der Kolk, and Peter Levine, in a talk moderated by Deb Dana, "Trauma and Safety in the Context of Current Day Issues," presentation at The Master Series, Oxford, England, August 31, 2023.

142 **Nearly a century ago:** Carl Jung, *The Portable Jung*, ed. Joseph Campbell (New York: Penguin Classics, 1971), 478.

143 **in early periods of Egyptian:** "Egyptian Mummies," Smithsonian, n.d., https://www.si.edu/spotlight/ancient-egypt/mummies; Rogerio Sousa, *Heart of Wisdom: Studies on the Heart Amulet in Ancient Egypt* (Oxford: British Archaeological Reports, 2011).

143 **"In the morning he was Khepri":** Garry J. Shaw, *Egyptian Myths: A Guide to the Ancient Gods and Legends* (London: Thames & Hudson, 2014), loc. 485.

143 **Amulets in the:** Metropolitan Museum of Art, "Heart Scarab of Hatnefer," n.d., https://www.metmuseum.org/art/collection/search/545146#:~:text

=The%20flat%20underside%20of%20a,30A%2C%20which%20was %20used%20here; E. A. Wallace Budge, trans., *The Egyptian Book of the Dead*, introduction by John Romer (London: Penguin Classics, 2008).

Chapter 6: Anchors: Story, Love, and Belonging

148 **The myth of P'an Ku:** Barbara C. Sproul, *Primal Myths: Creation Myths Around the World* (New York: HarperOne, 1979), 201.

148 **In Quiché Mayan:** Sproul, *Primal Myths*, 289.

148 **And from Greek and Roman:** Philip Matyszak, *The Greek and Roman Myths: A Guide to the Classical Stories* (London: Thames & Hudson, 2019), 10.

148 **"We sit here":** Homer, *The Iliad*, trans. Emily Wilson (New York: W. W. Norton & Company, 2023), 588–89.

150 **In an essay:** Adam Phillips, *Promises Promises* (London: Faber and Faber, 2000), 4–5.

150 **In the words:** Lionel Trilling, *The Liberal Imagination* (New York: Viking Press, 1950), 321.

150 **among children who:** Guilherme Brockington et al., "Storytelling Increases Oxytocin and Positive Emotions and Decreases Cortisol and Pain in Hospitalized Children," *Proceedings of the National Academy of Sciences* 118, no. 22 (June 1, 2021): e2018409118, https://doi.org/10.1073/pnas.2018409118.

151 **demonstrated the importance:** E.g., Kelly M. Christian, Sandra Russ, and Elizabeth J. Short, "Pretend Play Processes and Anxiety: Considerations for the Play Therapist," *International Journal of Play Therapy* 20, no. 4 (October 2011): 179–92, https://doi.org/10.1037/a0025324.

151 **"Mental illnesses are":** Rachel Aviv, *Strangers to Ourselves: Unsettled Minds and the Stories That Make Us* (New York: Farrar, Straus and Giroux, 2022), 22.

153 **Philip Matyszak writes:** Matyszak, *The Greek and Roman Myths*.

155 **And they found that parents':** Sachine Yoshida et al., "Infants Show Physiological Responses Specific to Parental Hugs," *iScience* 23, no. 4 (April 2020): 100996, https://doi.org/10.1016/j.isci.2020.100996.

155 **"love and attachment":** Inna Schneiderman et al., "Love Alters Autonomic Reactivity to Emotions," *Emotion* 11, no. 6 (2011): 1314–21, https://doi.org/10.1037/a0024090.

155 **researchers found that for adolescents:** Kenny Chiu, David M. Clark, and Eleanor Leigh, "Prospective Associations Between Peer Functioning and Social Anxiety in Adolescents: A Systematic Review and Meta-Analysis," *Journal of Affective Disorders* 279 (January 2021): 650–61, https://doi.org/10.1016/j.jad.2020.10.055.

155 **And a study on older:** Nirmala Lekhak et al., "The Primacy of Compassionate Love: Loneliness and Psychological Well-Being in Later Life," *Journal of Gerontological Nursing* 49, no. 4 (April 2023): 12–20, https://doi.org/10.3928/00989134-20230309-03.

155 **People who experience social anxiety:** Kit Casey et al., "Romantic Relationship Quality and Functioning for Individuals with Clinical and Sub-Clinical Social Anxiety: A Scoping Review," *Journal of Mental Health* (July 3, 2022): 1–29, https://doi.org/10.1080/09638237.2022.2091755.

156 **children who were observed to:** Francis Vergunst et al., "Behavior in Childhood Is Associated with Romantic Partnering Patterns in Adulthood," *Journal of Child Psychology and Psychiatry* 62, no. 7 (July 14, 2021): 842–52, https://doi.org/10.1111/jcpp.13329.

156 **They found that:** Eliora Porter et al., "Social Anxiety Disorder and Perceived Criticism in Intimate Relationships: Comparisons with Normal and Clinical Control Groups," *Behavior Therapy* 50, no. 1 (January 2019): 241–53, https://doi.org/10.1016/j.beth.2018.05.005.

156 **Loneliness is consistently:** Farhana Mann et al., "Loneliness and the Onset of New Mental Health Problems in the General Population," *Social Psychiatry and Psychiatric Epidemiology* 57, no. 11 (November 18, 2022): 2161–78, https://doi.org/10.1007/s00127-022-02261-7.

156 **By measuring these dimensions:** Joan Domènech-Abella et al., "Anxiety, Depression, Loneliness and Social Network in the Elderly: Longitudinal Associations from The Irish Longitudinal Study on Ageing (TILDA)," *Journal of Affective Disorders* 246 (March 2019): 82–88, https://doi.org/10.1016/j.jad.2018.12.043.

156 **the problems of loneliness:** Minhal Ahmed, Ivo Cerda, and Molly
Maloof, "Breaking the Vicious Cycle: The Interplay Between Loneliness,
Metabolic Illness, and Mental Health," *Frontiers in Psychiatry* 14 (March 8,
2023): https://doi.org/10.3389/fpsyt.2023.1134865; Domènech-Abella et al.,
"Anxiety, Depression, Loneliness and Social Network in the Elderly."

157 **They point to the work:** John Cacioppo and William Patrick, *Loneliness:
Human Nature and the Need for Social Connection* (New York: W. W.
Norton & Company, 2009), 17.

157 **surgeon general of:** Vivek H. Murthy, *Together: Loneliness, Health & What
Happens When We Find Connection* (London: Profile Books, 2021), 11.

157 **This process of self-regulation:** E.g., Stephen W. Porges, "Polyvagal Theory: A Biobehavioral Journey to Sociality," *Comprehensive Psychoneuroendocrinology* 7 (August 2021): 100069, https://doi.org/10.1016/j.cpnec.2021.100069.
Porges describes a facet of this process as "neuroception": "Polyvagal theory
proposes that the neural evaluation of risk and safety reflexively triggers
shifts in autonomic state without requiring conscious awareness."

158 **belonging during the hurricane:** Hannah C. Broos, Maria M. Llabre, and
Kiara R. Timpano, "Belonging Buffers the Impact of Cognitive Vulnerabil-
ities on Affective Symptoms," *Cognitive Therapy and Research* 46, no. 2
(April 26, 2022): 393–405, https://doi.org/10.1007/s10608-021-10267-9.

161 **In *Heart: A History*:** Sandeep Jauhar, *Heart: A History* (New York: Farrar,
Straus and Giroux, 2018), 24.

161 **Research consistently links takotsubo:** Arash Nayeri et al., "Psychiatric
Illness in Takotsubo (Stress) Cardiomyopathy: A Review," *Psychosomatics*
59, no. 3 (May 2018): 220–26, https://doi.org/10.1016/j.psym.2018.01.011.

162 **In a recently published paper:** Aaron H. Wasserman et al., "Oxytocin
Promotes Epicardial Cell Activation and Heart Regeneration after Cardiac
Injury," *Frontiers in Cell and Developmental Biology* 10 (September 30,
2022): 16, https://doi.org/10.3389/fcell.2022.985298.

Chapter 7: Interconnectedness

168 **We can look to Chinese medicine:** J. J. Y. Sung, "Acupuncture for Gastrointestinal Disorders: Myth or Magic," *Gut* 51, no. 5 (November 1, 2002):

617–19, https://doi.org/10.1136/gut.51.5.617; Robert Keith Wallace, "The Microbiome in Health and Disease from the Perspective of Modern Medicine and Ayurveda," *Medicina* 56, no. 9 (September 11, 2020): 462, https://doi.org/10.3390/medicina56090462.

168 **He points to the work:** Ian Miller, "The Gut–Brain Axis: Historical Reflections," *Microbial Ecology in Health and Disease* 29, no. 2 (November 23, 2018): 1542921, https://doi.org/10.1080/16512235.2018.1542921.

168 **in Victorian medicine:** Ian Miller, *A Modern History of the Stomach: Gastric Illness, Medicine and British Society, 1800–1950* (Abingdon: Oxfordshire: Routledge, 2011), 2.

171 **Scientists have consistently:** E.g., Gertjan Medema et al., "Presence of SARS-Coronavirus-2 RNA in Sewage and Correlation with Reported COVID-19 Prevalence in the Early Stage of the Epidemic in the Netherlands," *Environmental Science & Technology Letters* 7, no. 7 (July 14, 2020): 511–16, https://doi.org/10.1021/acs.estlett.0c00357; Jayaprakash Saththasivam et al., "COVID-19 (SARS-CoV-2) Outbreak Monitoring Using Wastewater-Based Epidemiology in Qatar," *Science of the Total Environment* 774 (June 2021): 145608, https://doi.org/10.1016/j.scitotenv.2021.145608; Kamila Zdenkova et al., "Monitoring COVID-19 Spread in Prague Local Neighborhoods Based on the Presence of SARS-CoV-2 RNA in Wastewater Collected throughout the Sewer Network," *Water Research* 216 (June 2022): 118343, https://doi.org/10.1016/j.watres.2022.118343.

171 **Over the past few decades:** Michael D. Gershon, *The Second Brain: A Groundbreaking New Understanding of Nervous Disorders of the Stomach and Intestine* (New York: Harper, 1998), iii.

172 **Gershon and colleague:** Michael D. Gershon and Kara Gross Margolis, "The Gut, Its Microbiome, and the Brain: Connections and Communications," *Journal of Clinical Investigation* 131, no. 18 (September 15, 2021): 1, https://doi.org/10.1172/JCI143768.

172 **The vast majority:** Natalie Terry and Kara Gross Margolis, "Serotonergic Mechanisms Regulating the GI Tract: Experimental Evidence and Therapeutic Relevance," 2016, 319–42, https://doi.org/10.1007/164_2016_103; Panida Sittipo et al., "The Function of Gut Microbiota in Immune-Related Neurological Disorders: A Review," *Journal of Neuroinflammation* 19, no. 1 (December 15, 2022): 154, https://doi.org/10.1186/s12974-022-02510-1.

172 **The microbiome refers:** "Microbiome," National Human Genome Research Institute, https://www.genome.gov/genetics-glossary/Microbiome.

173 **In *I Contain Multitudes*:** Ed Yong, *I Contain Multitudes: The Microbes Within Us and a Grander View of Life* (New York: HarperCollins, 2016), 17–18.

173 **not all babies are born:** Suchitra K. Hourigan, Maria Gloria Dominguez-Bello, and Noel T. Mueller, "Can Maternal-Child Microbial Seeding Interventions Improve the Health of Infants Delivered by Cesarean Section?," *Cell Host & Microbe* 30, no. 5 (May 2022): 607–11, https://doi.org /10.1016/j.chom.2022.02.014; Aneta Słabuszewska-Jóźwiak et al., "Pediatrics Consequences of Caesarean Section—A Systematic Review and Meta-Analysis," *International Journal of Environmental Research and Public Health* 17, no. 21 (October 31, 2020): 8031, https://doi.org/10.3390/ijerph 17218031.

174 **when comparing babies born:** Se Jin Song et al., "Naturalization of the Microbiota Developmental Trajectory of Cesarean-Born Neonates after Vaginal Seeding," *Med* 2, no. 8 (August 2021): 951–964.e5, https://doi.org /10.1016/j.medj.2021.05.003.

174 **as with so many aspects:** Hannah E. Laue, Modupe O. Coker, and Juliette C. Madan, "The Developing Microbiome from Birth to 3 Years: The Gut-Brain Axis and Neurodevelopmental Outcomes," *Frontiers in Pediatrics* 10 (March 7, 2022): https://doi.org/10.3389/fped.2022.815885.

174 **Our guts, too:** Laue, Coker, and Madan, "The Developing Microbiome from Birth to 3 Years."

175 **less gut microbiome diversity:** Hai-yin Jiang et al., "Altered Gut Microbiota Profile in Patients with Generalized Anxiety Disorder," *Journal of Psychiatric Research* 104 (September 2018): 130–36, https://doi.org/10.1016 /j.jpsychires.2018.07.007; Sun-Young Kim et al., "Association Between Gut Microbiota and Anxiety Symptoms: A Large Population-Based Study Examining Sex Differences," *Journal of Affective Disorders* 333 (July 2023): 21–29, https://doi.org/10.1016/j.jad.2023.04.003.

175 **One of these research teams:** Jiang et al., "Altered Gut Microbiota Profile in Patients with Generalized Anxiety Disorder."

175 **However, they did find:** Carra A. Simpson et al., "The Gut Microbiota in Anxiety and Depression—A Systematic Review," *Clinical Psychology Review* 83 (February 2021): 101943, https://doi.org/10.1016/j.cpr.2020.101943.

177 **Researchers found that:** Elena J. L. Coley et al., "Early Life Adversity Predicts Brain-Gut Alterations Associated with Increased Stress and Mood," *Neurobiology of Stress* 15 (November 2021): 100348, https://doi.org/10.1016/j.ynstr.2021.100348.

179 **anxiety and depression were linked to:** Keeley M. Fairbrass et al., "Bidirectional Brain–Gut Axis Effects Influence Mood and Prognosis in IBD: A Systematic Review and Meta-Analysis," *Gut* 71, no. 9 (November 1, 2021): 28, https://doi.org/10.1136/gutjnl-2021-325985.

179 **There are "shared pathogenic pathways":** Chris Eijsbouts et al., "Genome-Wide Analysis of 53,400 People with Irritable Bowel Syndrome Highlights Shared Genetic Pathways with Mood and Anxiety Disorders," *Nature Genetics* 53, no. 11 (November 5, 2021): 1543–52, https://doi.org/10.1038/s41588-021-00950-8.

180 **Fecal transplants, in:** Joshua Stripling and Martin Rodriguez, "Current Evidence in Delivery and Therapeutic Uses of Fecal Microbiota Transplantation in Human Diseases—Clostridium Difficile Disease and Beyond," *American Journal of the Medical Sciences* 356, no. 5 (November 2018): 424–32, https://doi.org/10.1016/j.amjms.2018.08.010.

180 **Research suggests that fecal transplants:** Jessica Emily Green et al., "Efficacy and Safety of Fecal Microbiota Transplantation for the Treatment of Diseases Other than *Clostridium Difficile* Infection: A Systematic Review and Meta-Analysis," *Gut Microbes* 12, no. 1 (November 9, 2020): 1854640, https://doi.org/10.1080/19490976.2020.1854640.

181 **Research, though in its very early stages:** E.g., Arthi Chinna Meyyappan et al., "Effect of Fecal Microbiota Transplant on Symptoms of Psychiatric Disorders: A Systematic Review," *BMC Psychiatry* 20, no. 1 (December 15, 2020): 299, https://doi.org/10.1186/s12888-020-02654-5; Yiming Meng, Jing Sun, and Guirong Zhang, "Pick Fecal Microbiota Transplantation to Enhance Therapy for Major Depressive Disorder," *Progress in Neuro-Psychopharmacology and Biological Psychiatry* 128 (January 2024): 110860, https://doi.org/10.1016/j.pnpbp.2023.110860.

181 **review of research on fecal transplants:** Chinna Meyyappan et al., "Effect of Fecal Microbiota Transplant on Symptoms of Psychiatric Disorders."

181 **What's more, this review:** Chinna Meyyappan et al., "Effect of Fecal Microbiota Transplant on Symptoms of Psychiatric Disorders."

181 **the same research team:** Arthi Chinna Meyyappan, Evan Forth, and Roumen Milev, "Microbial Ecosystem Therapeutic-2 Intervention in People with Major Depressive Disorder and Generalized Anxiety Disorder: Phase 1, Open-Label Study," *Interactive Journal of Medical Research* 11, no. 1 (January 21, 2022): e32234, https://doi.org/10.2196/32234.

182 **studies with human subjects:** Chinna Meyyappan et al., "Effect of Fecal Microbiota Transplant on Symptoms of Psychiatric Disorders."

183 **In particular, they point to:** Penny M. Kris-Etherton et al., "Nutrition and Behavioral Health Disorders: Depression and Anxiety," *Nutrition Reviews* 79, no. 3 (February 11, 2021): 247–60, https://doi.org/10.1093/nutrit/nuaa025.

183 **Some scientists even view anxiety:** Nicholas G. Norwitz and Uma Naidoo, "Nutrition as Metabolic Treatment for Anxiety," *Frontiers in Psychiatry* 12 (February 12, 2021): 2, https://doi.org/10.3389/fpsyt.2021.598119.

183 **They argue that:** Norwitz and Naidoo, "Nutrition as Metabolic Treatment for Anxiety," 2.

185 **Evidence is mixed at best:** Jaqueline S. Generoso et al., "The Role of the Microbiota-Gut-Brain Axis in Neuropsychiatric Disorders," *Brazilian Journal of Psychiatry* 43, no. 3 (June 2021): 293–305, https://doi.org/10.1590/1516-4446-2020-0987.

185 **no meaningful changes:** A. Zagórska et al., "From Probiotics to Psychobiotics—the Gut-Brain Axis in Psychiatric Disorders," *Beneficial Microbes* 11, no. 8 (December 2, 2020): 717–32, https://doi.org/10.3920/BM2020.0063.

185 **another review of research on probiotic use:** Sabrina Mörkl et al., "Probiotics and the Microbiota-Gut-Brain Axis: Focus on Psychiatry," *Current Nutrition Reports* 9, no. 3 (September 13, 2020): 171–82, https://doi.org/10.1007/s13668-020-00313-5.

186 Reading in this field: E.g., Tommaso Ballarini et al., "Mediterranean Diet, Alzheimer Disease Biomarkers, and Brain Atrophy in Old Age," *Neurology* 96, no. 24 (June 15, 2021): e2920–32, https://doi.org/10.1212/WNL.0000000000012067.

Chapter 8: Trust and Agency

195 Research in psychology and political science: E.g., Michael H. Connors and Matthew M. Large, "Calibrating Violence Risk Assessments for Uncertainty," *General Psychiatry* 36, no. 2 (April 28, 2023): e100921, https://doi.org/10.1136/gpsych-2022-100921; Barbara Mellers et al., "Identifying and Cultivating Superforecasters as a Method of Improving Probabilistic Predictions," *Perspectives on Psychological Science* 10, no. 3 (May 18, 2015): 267–81, https://doi.org/10.1177/1745691615577794; Phillip Tetlock and Dan Gardner, *Superforecasting: The Art and Science of Prediction* (New York: Crown, 2015).

196 Nor are we very good: Maya A. Pilin, "The Past of Predicting the Future: A Review of the Multidisciplinary History of Affective Forecasting," *History of the Human Sciences* 34, no. 3–4 (July 28, 2021): 290–306, https://doi.org/10.1177/0952695120976330.

197 He chronicles the work of: As cited in Sam Knight, "The Psychiatrist Who Believed People Could Tell the Future," *New Yorker*, February 25, 2019, 15.

198 In Knight's words: Knight, "The Psychiatrist Who Believed People Could Tell the Future," 17. In 2022, Sam Knight published a book on the same topic titled *The Premonitions Bureau: A True Story* (London: Faber and Faber, 2022).

202 tend to perceive the risk: E.g., Catherine A. Hartley and Elizabeth A. Phelps, "Anxiety and Decision-Making," *Biological Psychiatry* 72, no. 2 (July 2012): 113–18, https://doi.org/10.1016/j.biopsych.2011.12.027; Jon K. Maner and Norman B. Schmidt, "The Role of Risk Avoidance in Anxiety," *Behavior Therapy* 37, no. 2 (June 2006): 181–89, https://doi.org/10.1016/j.beth.2005.11.003.

203 "reliance on affect in situations of risk and uncertainty": Martina Raue and Elisabeth Schneider, "Psychological Perspectives on Perceived Safety: Zero-Risk Bias, Feelings and Learned Carelessness" in *Perceived Safety: A*

Multidisciplinary Perspective, eds. Martina Raue, Bernard Streicher, and Eva Lermer (Cham, Switzerland: Springer, 2019): 61–81, https://doi.org/10 .1007/978-3-030-11456-5_5; Paul Slovic, *The Feeling of Risk: New Perspectives on Risk Perception* (London and Washington, DC: Earthscan, 2010); Paul Slovic and Ellen Peters, "Risk Perception and Affect," *Current Directions in Psychological Science* 15, no. 6 (December 2006): 322–25, https://doi.org /10.1111/j.1467-8721.2006.00461.x.

203 **a tendency to make:** E.g., Sonia J. Bishop and Christopher Gagne, "Anxiety, Depression, and Decision Making: A Computational Perspective," *Annual Review of Neuroscience* 41, no. 1 (July 8, 2018): 371–88, https://doi .org/10.1146/annurev-neuro-080317-062007.

204 **study that was conducted in mid-2020:** Tosin Philip Oyetunji et al., "COVID-19-Related Risk Perception, Anxiety and Protective Behaviours among Nigerian Adults: A Cross-Sectional Study," *Journal of Public Health* (March 11, 2021): https://doi.org/10.1007/s10389-021-01502-4.

204 **Another study, conducted in Italy:** Sofia Tagini et al., "Attachment, Personality and Locus of Control: Psychological Determinants of Risk Perception and Preventive Behaviors for COVID-19," *Frontiers in Psychology* 12 (July 9, 2021): https://doi.org/10.3389/fpsyg.2021.634012.

205 **Rather, they tend to feel:** E.g., Johanna H. M. Hovenkamp-Hermelink et al., "Differential Associations of Locus of Control with Anxiety, Depression and Life-Events: A Five-Wave, Nine-Year Study to Test Stability and Change," *Journal of Affective Disorders* 253 (June 2019): 26–34, https://doi .org/10.1016/j.jad.2019.04.005.

205 **Our sense of where control:** Hovenkamp-Hermelink et al., "Differential Associations of Locus of Control with Anxiety, Depression and Life-Events."

206 **well established that OCD:** Ryan Mitchell, Donncha Hanna, and Kevin F. W. Dyer, "Modelling OCD: A Test of the Inflated Responsibility Model," *Behavioural and Cognitive Psychotherapy* 48, no. 3 (May 31, 2020): 327–40, https://doi.org/10.1017/S1352465819000675; Paul Salkovskis et al., "Multiple Pathways to Inflated Responsibility Beliefs in Obsessional Problems: Possible Origins and Implications for Therapy and Research," *Behaviour Research and Therapy* 37, no. 11 (November 1999): 1055–72, https://doi.org/10.1016/S0005 -7967(99)00063-7; Paul M. Salkovskis, "Obsessional-Compulsive Problems:

A Cognitive-Behavioural Analysis," *Behaviour Research and Therapy* 23, no. 5 (1985): 571–83, https://doi.org/10.1016/0005-7967(85)90105-6.

206 I think again of the: Stanley Rachman and Ray Hodgson, *Obsessions and Compulsions* (Englewood Cliffs, NJ: Prentice-Hall, 1980), 252.

206 Research shows that an inflated: E.g., Andrea Pozza and Davide Dèttore, "The Specificity of Inflated Responsibility Beliefs to OCD: A Systematic Review and Meta-Analysis of Published Cross-Sectional Case-Control Studies," *Research in Psychology and Behavioral Sciences* 2, no. 4 (November 1, 2014): 75–85, https://doi.org/10.12691/rpbs-2-4-1; Yoshinori Sugiura and Brian Fisak, "Inflated Responsibility in Worry and Obsessive Thinking," *International Journal of Cognitive Therapy* 12, no. 2 (June 1, 2019): 97–108, https://doi.org/10.1007/s41811-019-00041-x.

206 It bears repeating that anxiety: Debra A. Bangasser and Amelia Cuarenta, "Sex Differences in Anxiety and Depression: Circuits and Mechanisms," *Nature Reviews Neuroscience* 22, no. 11 (November 20, 2021): 674–84, https://doi.org/10.1038/s41583-021-00513-0; Ronald C. Kessler et al., "Twelve-Month and Lifetime Prevalence and Lifetime Morbid Risk of Anxiety and Mood Disorders in the United States," *International Journal of Methods in Psychiatric Research* 21, no. 3 (September 2012): 169–84, https://doi.org/10.1002/mpr.1359.

206 when it comes to GAD: Pablo J. Olivares-Olivares et al., "Obsessive Beliefs and Uncertainty in Obsessive Compulsive and Related Patients," *International Journal of Clinical and Health Psychology* 22, no. 3 (September 2022): 100316, https://doi.org/10.1016/j.ijchp.2022.100316.

Chapter 9: Sublimation and Subversion

213 Is every wall: The phrase "every wall is a door" is typically attributed to Ralph Waldo Emerson, but appears as "every wall is a gate." See Ralph Waldo Emerson, *The Complete Works of Ralph Waldo Emerson: Natural History of Intellect, and Other Papers [vol. 12]* (Boston and New York: Houghton Mifflin, 1903), 442.

215 The American Psychological: G. R. VandenBos, ed., *APA Dictionary of Psychology* (Washington, DC: American Psychological Association, 2015).

216 higher scores on a measure of resilience: Mariela Loreto Lara-Cabrera et al., "The Mediating Role of Resilience in the Relationship Between

Perceived Stress and Mental Health," *International Journal of Environmental Research and Public Health* 18, no. 18 (September 16, 2021): 9762, https://doi .org/10.3390/ijerph18189762.

217 **Cal Flyn describes:** Cal Flyn, *Islands of Abandonment: Nature Rebounding in the Post-Human Landscape* (New York: Viking, 2021), 323.

219 **And we can develop resilience:** E.g., Sadhbh Joyce et al., "Road to Resilience: A Systematic Review and Meta-Analysis of Resilience Training Programmes and Interventions," *British Medical Journal Open* 8, no. 6 (June 14, 2018): e017858, https://doi.org/10.1136/bmjopen-2017-017858; Steven M. Southwick and Dennis S. Charney, *Resilience: The Science of Mastering Life's Greatest Challenges* (Cambridge: Cambridge University Press, 2018).

219 **Instead, resilience is:** E.g., Esther Mesman, Annabel Vreeker, and Manon Hillegers, "Resilience and Mental Health in Children and Adolescents: An Update of the Recent Literature and Future Directions," *Current Opinion in Psychiatry* 34, no. 6 (November 2021): 586–92, https://doi.org/10.1097/YCO .0000000000000741; Schiele and Domschke, "Epigenetics at the Crossroads Between Genes, Environment and Resilience in Anxiety Disorders"; Michael Ungar and Linda Theron, "Resilience and Mental Health: How Multisystemic Processes Contribute to Positive Outcomes," *The Lancet Psychiatry* 7, no. 5 (May 2020): 441–48, https://doi.org/10.1016/S2215-0366(19)30434-1.

219 **"Resilience can be broadly defined":** Ann S. Masten, "Global Perspectives on Resilience in Children and Youth," *Child Development* 85, no. 1 (January 2014): 6–20, https://doi.org/10.1111/cdev.12205.

220 **They remind us that despite:** Research on ritual tends to fall under the purview of anthropology, and in this arena, rituals have been defined with great specificity. When I refer to rituals, I use the term in its broader, more colloquial sense. For more on rituals as understood from an anthropological standpoint, see, for instance, the excellent work of anthropologist Catherine Bell: Catherine Bell, *Ritual: Perspectives and Dimensions* (Oxford: Oxford University Press, 1997); Catherine Bell, *Ritual Theory, Ritual Practice* (Oxford: Oxford University Press, 1992).

221 **People attended either communal:** Sarah J. Charles et al., "United on Sunday: The Effects of Secular Rituals on Social Bonding and Affect," *PLOS ONE* 16, no. 1 (January 27, 2021): e0242546, https://doi.org/10.1371 /journal.pone.0242546.

222 one of the central aspects: E.g., Allison L. Baier, Alexander C. Kline, and Norah C. Feeny, "Therapeutic Alliance as a Mediator of Change: A Systematic Review and Evaluation of Research," *Clinical Psychology Review* 82 (December 2020): 101921, https://doi.org/10.1016/j.cpr.2020.101921; Christoph Flückiger et al., "The Alliance in Adult Psychotherapy: A Meta-Analytic Synthesis," *Psychotherapy* 55, no. 4 (December 2018): 316–40, https://doi.org/10.1037/pst0000172; Jeremy D. Safran, J. Christopher Muran, and Catherine Eubanks-Carter, "Repairing Alliance Ruptures," *Psychotherapy* 48, no. 1 (2011): 80–87, https://doi.org/10.1037/a0022140.

222 Porges writes, "Resiliency": Stephen W. Porges, "Polyvagal Theory: A Science of Safety," *Frontiers in Integrative Neuroscience* 16 (May 10, 2022): 11, https://doi.org/10.3389/fnint.2022.871227.

223 all the participants: Alia J. Crum and Ellen J. Langer, "Mind-Set Matters," *Psychological Science* 18, no. 2 (February 6, 2007): 165–71, https://doi.org/10.1111/j.1467-9280.2007.01867.x.

223 The placebome, a term: Kathryn T. Hall, Joseph Loscalzo, and Ted J. Kaptchuk, "Genetics and the Placebo Effect: The Placebome," *Trends in Molecular Medicine* 21, no. 5 (May 2015): 285–94, https://doi.org/10.1016/j.molmed.2015.02.009.

223 Hall's research points: Kathryn T. Hall, Joseph Loscalzo, and Ted Kaptchuk, "Pharmacogenomics and the Placebo Response," *ACS Chemical Neuroscience* 9, no. 4 (April 18, 2018): 633–35, https://doi.org/10.1021/acschemneuro.8b00078; Kathryn T. Hall et al., "Catechol-O-Methyltransferase Val158met Polymorphism Predicts Placebo Effect in Irritable Bowel Syndrome," *PLOS One* 7, no. 10 (October 23, 2012): e48135, https://doi.org/10.1371/journal.pone.0048135.

224 "While positive expectations": Hailey E. Yetman et al., "What Do Placebo and Nocebo Effects Have to Do with Health Equity? The Hidden Toll of Nocebo Effects on Racial and Ethnic Minority Patients in Clinical Care," *Frontiers in Psychology* 12 (December 23, 2021): 788230, https://doi.org/10.3389/fpsyg.2021.788230.

228 Through this lens: Elizabeth L. Auchincloss and Eslee Samberg, eds., *Psychoanalytic Terms & Concepts* (New Haven and London: American Psychoanalytic Association and Yale University Press, 2012), 252.

229 definitions of subversion: "Subversion, n. Meanings, Etymology and More," OED Online, Oxford University Press, 2022, https://www.oed.com /dictionary/subversion_n.

229 Ruth Ozeki, the writer: Ezra Klein (host) and Ruth Ozeki (guest), "What We Gain by Enchanting the Objects in Our Lives/Learning to Listen to the Voices That Only You Hear," *The Ezra Klein Show* (podcast), *New York Times*, January 25, 2022.